Living with Multiple Sclerosis

I0130643

Connecting theory, research and intervention, *Living with Multiple Sclerosis* offers an effective, innovative and comprehensive group-based psychological support intervention specifically aimed at people newly diagnosed with multiple sclerosis (LiMS).

The book explains the theoretical foundations of the intervention, based on developmental psychology in the life cycle, and considering the illness as a challenge to personal development. It analyzes the psychological aspects addressed in the intervention: the redefinition of identity, the sense of coherence, the sense of self-efficacy in coping with the illness, the emotional experiences, the relationship between thoughts and emotions and the effective communication strategies. Describing all session-by-session activities that are carried out in group meetings, it allows for timely replication of the intervention, while still accommodating possible adaptations to specific local and cultural contexts. It gives a concrete, positive perspective of personal fulfilment for people living with MS. Furthermore, it illustrates the central role of research in the project and presents new perspectives in research and intervention focused on parenthood.

The book is valuable reading for psychologists, researchers and health professionals such as occupational or rehabilitation therapists working with people with MS, as well as students specializing in clinical, health or developmental psychology.

Silvia Bonino, psychologist (M.A., Ph.D.) and psychotherapist, is Emeritus Professor of Developmental and Educational Psychology at the Department of Psychology at the University of Turin (Italy). She is the author of *Nature and Culture in Intimate Partner Violence: Sex, Love and Equality* (Routledge, 2018) and *Coping with Chronic Illness: Theories, Issues and Lived Experiences* (Routledge, 2021).

Martina Borghi, psychologist (M.A.) and psychotherapist, works at CReSM (Regional Referral Centre for Multiple Sclerosis), AOU San Luigi Gonzaga Hospital, Orbassano, Torino (Italy), and collaborates with AISM (Italian SM Society).

Emanuela Calandri, psychologist (M.A., Ph.D.), is Associate Professor of Developmental and Educational Psychology at the Department of Psychology at the University of Turin (Italy).

Federica Graziano, psychologist (M.A., Ph.D.), works at the Department of Psychology at the University of Turin (Italy).

Living with Multiple Sclerosis

A Group-Based Psychological Support
Intervention for Newly Diagnosed People with
MS (LiMS)

**Silvia Bonino, Martina Borghi,
Emanuela Calandri and Federica Graziano**

Routledge
Taylor & Francis Group

LONDON AND NEW YORK

Designed cover image: Getty Images via Eoneren

First published 2026
by Routledge
4 Park Square, Milton Park, Abingdon, Oxon OX14 4RN

and by Routledge
605 Third Avenue, New York, NY 10158

Routledge is an imprint of the Taylor & Francis Group, an informa business

© 2026 Silvia Bonino, Martina Borghi, Emanuela Calandri
and Federica Graziano

Published in Italian by Edizioni Centro Studi Erickson 2021. *Vivere con la sclerosi multipla.* © 2021 by Edizioni Centro Studi Erickson S.p.A., Trento (Italy). All rights reserved
www.erickson.it
www.erickson.international

Translated by Sheri Dorn Giarmoleo

The right of Silvia Bonino, Martina Borghi, Emanuela Calandri, and Federica Graziano to be identified as authors of this work has been asserted in accordance with sections 77 and 78 of the Copyright, Designs and Patents Act 1988.

This translation is made with the contribution of the Cosso Foundation (S. Secondo di Pinerolo, Torino, Italy)

British Library Cataloguing-in-Publication Data
A catalogue record for this book is available from the British Library

Library of Congress Cataloging-in-Publication Data
Names: Bonino, Silvia author | Borghi, Martina author |
Calandri, Emanuela author | Graziano, Federica author
Title: Living with multiple sclerosis : a group-based psychological support intervention for newly diagnosed people with MS (LiMS) / Silvia Bonino, Martina Borghi, Emanuela Calandri, Federica Graziano.
Other titles: Vivere con la sclerosi multipla. English
Description: Abingdon, Oxon ; New York, NY : Routledge, 2026. |
Published in Italian by Edizioni Centro Studi Erickson 2021. Vivere con la sclerosi multipla. | Includes bibliographical references and index.
Identifiers: LCCN 2025009876 (print) | LCCN 2025009877 (ebook) |
ISBN 9781032777023 hardback | ISBN 9781032776965 paperback |
ISBN 9781003484400 ebook
Subjects: LCSH: Multiple sclerosis | Group psychotherapy |
Multiple sclerosis--Patients--Mental health services |
Multiple sclerosis--Patients--Mental health
Classification: LCC RC377 .B6613 2026 (print) |
LCC RC377 (ebook) LC record available at https://lccn.loc.gov/2025009876
LC ebook record available at https://lccn.loc.gov/2025009877

ISBN: 978-1-032-77702-3 (hbk)
ISBN: 978-1-032-77696-5 (pbk)
ISBN: 978-1-003-48440-0 (ebk)

DOI: 10.4324/9781003484400

Typeset in Times New Roman
by KnowledgeWorks Global Ltd.

Contents

Presentation

This book presents a psychological support intervention aimed at people with multiple sclerosis (MS), particularly with a primary focus on those who have been recently diagnosed. Implemented since 2009, it is the fruit of the ongoing collaboration between the Cosso Foundation (San Secondo di Pinerolo, Turin, Italy), the Regional Reference Center for Multiple Sclerosis (CReSM) of the S. Luigi Hospital in Orbassano (Turin, Italy), the Department of Psychology of the University of Turin (Italy). This intervention program is integrated with research work, aimed at evaluating its effectiveness and deepening the theoretical constructs that underlie its scope.

The publication in English is a response to the need of the international community, considering it is estimated that today 2.8 million people in the world live with this disease, hosting a huge impact on their lives. Consequently, the need for psychological support is deeply felt, but unfortunately, it often goes unmet. Here, there is a possibility of knowing in detail the intervention implemented, in its close connection with theory and research, so that those who treat people with MS can include it in the normal therapeutic activity of their clinical center.

It is our hope that professionals who dedicate themselves to the care of people with MS will be able to find in this book a well-founded help in their work, which may alternately inspire those who treat people with other chronic diseases.

Maria Luisa Cosso Eynard
Cosso Foundation President

Introduction

This book aims to describe the research and group psychological intervention pro-ject for people who have recently been diagnosed with multiple sclerosis (MS); its theoretical foundations are explained, the activities carried out are described, the developments and in-depth analyses derived from it, and the materials used are provided. The text is divided into five chapters and six appendices.

In the first chapter, the history of the project is illustrated, and its fundamental characteristics, specific features and innovative aspects are presented.The second chapter sets out the theoretical basis of the project. Starting from the conception of illness as a challenge to the individual's development throughout their lifespan, it considers the psychological aspects central to adaptation to one's illness, addressed in the intervention: the redefinition of identity, the sense of coherence, the sense of self-efficacy in coping with the illness and in managing symptoms, the emotional experiences, the relationship between thought and emotions and the effective com-munication strategies.

The third chapter describes in detail the group intervention implemented. In the chapter and in the appendices, traces of the meetings and materials used are made available, together with insights and suggestions for those who would like to pro-pose the intervention in their own care contexts.

The fourth chapter illustrates the central role of research in the project, as a tool that holds theory and intervention together in a circular process. It presents the results of the intervention evaluation, and an in-depth examination of some aspects still little investigated in the literature. In the chapter, appendices are research tools that can be used, subject to citation of the source, by those who intend to implement this intervention and at the same time evaluate its progress and effectiveness.

The fifth chapter presents some developments in our research and intervention work focused on the topic of MS and parenthood. The topic is addressed from two perspectives: that of the parent with a young adult child with MS and that of the parent who is ill himself. For both cases, theoretical and research insights are presented, and two pilot experiences of psychological support intervention are illustrated.

The appendices contain the materials used, the questionnaires and the observa-tion grid, as well as participants' testimonies. The appendices form an integral part of this volume not only to gain a close insight into the operational aspects of the intervention pathway but also to facilitate its implementation in other contexts.

Appendix 1 presents the handout, complete with materials for each meeting, to be distributed to participants. The photos shown are those we used and should be considered as an example to be adapted to the individual project context.

Appendix 2 collects the testimonies of the participants on the topics covered in each meeting. Their words allow us to capture in-depth and in a direct way their personal experiences. Again, the photos should be considered as an example to be adapted to the individual project contexts.

Appendix 3 proposes the instrument used to observe the groups, to record the characteristics and specific dynamics of each of them during each meeting.

In Appendices 4 and 5, we propose the two questionnaires (*Me and My Life* and *My Point of View*) used to evaluate the intervention process.

The volume concludes with Appendix 6, a collection of our scientific production related to the project, to allow for the in-depth examination of certain aspects, in the connection and circularity between research and intervention.

1 The history of the project and its characteristics

Silvia Bonino

The history of the project

The importance of the person

The research and intervention project dedicated to people who have recently received the diagnosis of multiple sclerosis (MS), presented in this book, owes its conception and implementation above all to the people who, in various capacities, have participated in it in recent years. We would like to underscore this because people are the determining variable in the success of a therapeutic intervention or research project, in this as in other cases, and not just good theories or good methodologies. The latter are not abstract entities, but are embodied in concrete people, who use thought and scientific knowledge but, at the same time, experience emotions, experience feelings, and establish significant social relationships. People who study, reflect on scientific models, imagine innovative solutions, beyond consolidated habits. It is from their thinking rationality that theoretical models and scientific methodologies derive, while it is from their affections, and in particular from their empathic sharing, there is the drive to know and act to alleviate the suffering, not only physical but also psychological, of the people affected by MS.

There are many people who brought this project to life and guaranteed its continuity over time.

The author of this chapter has chosen to write, because in me there is a fusion between psychological sciences and the personal experience of illness. When, over 25 years ago, I was diagnosed with MS which would radically change my existence, I asked myself how psychology, to which I had dedicated my life, could help me deal with this new condition full of unknowns. The fruit of that reflection was published in 2006 in the book *Mille fili mi legano qui. Vivere la malattia* (the second edition of which was released in 2019 and the English translation *Coping with chronic illness. Theories, issues and lived experiences* in 2021). The book is rightly defined as scientific and testimony, because it combines rigorous psychological reflection with the daily experience of the illness, in the experience of those who live it every day in its different aspects. This dual role made me a privileged witness, despite placing me in a very uncomfortable position.

DOI: 10.4324/9781003484400-1

The publication of the book was the starting point for numerous meetings with other people suffering from MS or other chronic diseases. It was these meetings and these people that gave the push to go beyond a simple book. In fact, there was a strong need to intervene to give sick people the tools to cope with the illness, in their daily lives, with the means that psychology had long ago identified as useful.

A decisive role was played by the people who participated in the intervention groups in recent years. They were not the passive recipients of an intervention; on the contrary, their active participation gave the push to continue and made it possible to carry out theoretical and methodological research work together, which led to the refinement and improvement of the intervention itself over time, also opening up, as we will see, new areas of in-depth analysis. They are the participants in the groups who, with their effort, commitment and participation, have allowed this project to come to fruition and improve. It is to these people, of all ages and from all backgrounds, who did not allow themselves to be defeated by suffering, but who continued to strive to give meaning to their lives, with difficulty but with equal determination, that this project owes its realization and its continuity.

Alongside them, there are those who believed in the project when it was only on paper and was struggling to get started because it appeared to many of the interlocutors to whom it was proposed as too new, too ambitious, not sufficiently evaluated. Since no initiative can be implemented without organizational involvement and without concrete support, in particular economic, the project owes its implementation first and foremost to the CReSM (Regional Reference Center for Multiple Sclerosis) of the AOU S. Luigi of Orbassano (Turin) and to the Cosso Foundation of S. Secondo di Pinerolo (Turin), to which was added the Department of Psychology of the University of Turin. These entities are not just acronyms, but are first and foremost people, who more than 15 years ago had faith in the project and invested human and economic resources in it: the CReSM by making its clinical structure available, the Cosso Foundation by financing the project and hosting the activities in the Miradolo Castle and the Department of Psychology by offering its own research facilities.

The collaboration between these diverse entities, both public and private, have continued through the years; this is most rare. It is thanks to their profound commitment to overcoming critical moments and demonstrating great strength that secured the continuity of this project.

Facing the necessity of psychological intervention

Psychological interventions concerning MS, in particular for those recently diagnosed, are basically lacking, not only lacking, but more often than not, are non-existent in relation to all chronic illnesses. In the first place, this derives from a cultural fracture, yet to be understood in the relationship between body and psyche, which directly reflects the educational formation of healthcare professionals. Even cutting-edge institutions providing care for individuals with chronic illness continue to completely ignore the psychological aspects of one having a chronic illness, as if this has no effect on the treatment of the illness that has struck the body of a person. Imagine the adherence to treatments, strictly connected to the modalities of psychological adjustment.

The second reason, linked to the first, is the chronicity of the illness itself. There is a lack of understanding that a chronic illness accompanies a person in every aspect of their existence, inescapably capturing entirely one's life, hence the totality of the person and their social relationships. There is no acute phase where a patient's body is treated, and the person is able to live life as before, closing a temporary parenthesis that leaves little or nothing in its wake. There is, on the contrary, a permanent condition that, as in the case of MS, is given to a progressively worsening condition with heavy consequences to one's entire existence.

The inception of this project therefore began from observing the pressing need for psychological interventions, yet at the same time completely absent. Psychological interventions are necessary clearly because chronic illness is exactly that, lifelong – posing its daily challenges. Increasingly necessary, because after the diagnosis, individuals must seek tools to deal with their situation in the best way possible without added suffering, without losing time, attempting to learn effective strategies in the arduous path of personal development. There is no one strategy that lasts forever, given the continuous evolution of chronic illness, but providing psychological interventions furnishes a strong basis for adapting to one's evolving future.

From a theoretical point of view, chronic illnesses are considered a great non-normative challenge to personal development; on a practical level, there is the necessity to propose psychological intervention to all those who are recently diagnosed with MS. The objective is to make this intervention a normal part of therapeutic practice in centers dedicated to the treatment of MS, together with pharmacological therapies. We are well aware that this is not easy, due to cultural and institutional resistance on the part of the healthcare system, which often claims there are very limited economic resources to provide such services. In addition, there is also a sense of resistance that comes from the patients themselves for the cultural reasons described above. Regardless, it remains an indispensable objective, in a situation in which not only chronic disease in general is on the increase, but specifically diagnoses are increasingly early and numerous, due to greater diagnostic precision. The road is certainly long and with this book we wish to give our contribution to achieving a difficult but not impossible goal; we cannot continue to delude ourselves that we are truly treating the ill, while ignoring their psyche.

A human, therapeutic and scientific adventure

The implementation of this project involves a simultaneous adventure of the following three inextricably linked components: human, therapeutic and scientific.

Why do we define it as an adventure? Despite the existing rigorous programs, meeting real people invariably introduces unexpected new elements that must be taken into consideration! We knew where we were starting from, what we wanted to achieve and by what means, while being mindful of the many uncontrolled variables that exist in relation to the complexities of a person's life experiences. All of this constitutes a challenge for those who lead the groups: (given the distinct aspects of each group) due to the relationships that are created with the arbitrary presence of different personalities, although, as we will see, quite homogeneous in age. But even the evaluation of the intervention itself is put to the test, because it is necessary to continually ask ourselves what needs to be modified as this process progresses through the years.

It is a human adventure, wherein the interaction and views explored have enriched not only the group participants but all of us, members of the working group and organizers. The determination and strength of the participants within their daily struggles were encouraging to continue moving ahead, prompting for all a great life lesson.

It is a therapeutic adventure because there is a documented benefit for chronically ill persons who participate. In particular, an important benefit for those who, like the person who has recently received their diagnosis, find themselves in a moment of overwhelming difficulty and urgently need not suffer unnecessarily, to not waste time and energy, and to begin their life journey engaging with insightful methods and useful strategies as their illness demands.

The benefits have been evaluated with the tools of science, despite the challenges of doing psychological intervention research in a situation in which participants continue to lead their normal daily lives. This is a critically important aspect; from the beginning through a number of years, we always want to evaluate whether a group intervention project as we conceived and structured it would work, while considering how it could be more effective. It is therefore a scientific adventure, with different objectives: the evaluation of the project's effectiveness, both in the initial phase and when fully operational, the differentiation between the comparison group and the intervention group, the consistent evaluation of the methods of carrying out the project itself – for any changes or adjustments, the in-depth analysis of some basic psychological issues which allow for the construction of new evaluation tools.

Introductory information on the disease we are addressing is reported in Box 1.1.

Box 1.1   Some information about multiple sclerosis

MS is a chronic inflammatory and neurodegenerative disease of the central nervous system. The pathogenetic causes are unknown, but their autoimmune nature has been ascertained, which manifests itself on a genetic basis interacting with environmental factors. Immune cells trigger an aberrant inflammatory process which causes demyelination of the axons and slowing the conduction of nerve impulses, causing a degeneration of the central nervous system and permanent neuronal damage. Demyelination is multifocal and the symptoms are accordingly polymorphic (such as fatigue, balance disorders, motor difficulties, spasticity and urinary disorders).

The disease occurs mainly between the ages of 20 and 30, while it becomes rare after the age of 50. The women are affected more than men, in a ratio of 3:1.

There are 2.9 million people living with MS worldwide. Throughout the world, geographical distribution and prevalence are heterogeneous. The prevalence increases as one moves away in the two hemispheres, from the equator.

The disease presents with *different modes of evolution*, and the clinical course is variable and unpredictable. The first and most frequent form of MS (relapsing remitting multiple sclerosis – RRMS: 85% of cases) is characterized by acute phases followed by remissions of symptoms more or less complete, for periods of different durations; after a variable number of years, this form becomes mostly progressive (secondary progressive multiple sclerosis – SPMS), worsening without evident flare-ups. The second form (primary progressive multiple sclerosis – PPMS: 10% of cases) is characterized from the beginning by progression, without attacks of disease, while a third form, a minority (5%), presents both progression and flare-ups (relapsing progressive multiple sclerosis – RPMS). The diagnosis is based on clinical evidence and data from magnetic resonance imaging (MRI).

There are currently no curative treatments. The treatment of flare-ups mainly uses corticosteroids. Immunomodulatory therapies have been developed in recent decades capable of modifying the course of the disease (disease-modifying therapy – DMT) reducing the relapses and progression of disability for RRMS, while other forms of treatment are in experimentation.

The tool most used by neurologists for the evaluation of disability progression is the EDSS scale (Expanded Disability Status Scale; Kurtzke, 1983), with a scale from 0 to 10.

Due to its characteristics, MS has a strong psychological impact and very high human, health and social costs.

Characteristics of the project, its specifications and innovative aspects

Theoretical foundation

The project is characterized by having strong theoretical bases, which come from developmental psychology and health psychology. Developmental psychology will be explored in depth in Chapter 2; the basic concept considers illness as a challenge that can be faced, although difficult and non-normative, it does not impede the development of the person in their life cycle with illness. Also from developmental psychology comes the choice to consider crucial aspects for the development of the person such as identity, search for meaning, and the effective realization of significant objectives (Bonino, 2021). From health psychology, comes the attention paid to other aspects, such as the management of stress and symptoms, emotions, and their relationships with thought and communication.

The importance of theory must be underlined, because it is one of the strong points of the project in contrast with the tendency, unfortunately widespread today, to "do something" or apply pre-packaged methods of intervention that are fashionable, void of cultural sensibility, meaning without having a clear awareness of either the theoretical basis or the validity of what is being done. In line with a rigorous conception of psychological science, the project started from a very in-depth theoretical analysis. Even if it is understandable, in a situation in which psychological interventions are often absent or severely lacking, that psychologists are moved by the desire to intervene, one cannot but deprecate the temptation to act without sufficient theoretical bases, the only ones that can guide the choice of a valid intervention methodology, consistent with one's objectives. Fashions cannot guide the choice of interventions.

The theoretical premise was continuously compared, both in the start of the project and in its development, with the lived experiences of the participants. It is in the synergistic relationship between theory and personal experience that this project developed. However, it must be underscored that personal experience, alone, without rigorous reflection and a timely comparison with a theoretical framework capable of giving meaning, would have been useless and misleading, considering experiencing does not in itself mean knowing.

The strong theoretical reference is even more necessary when entering partially or completely unexplored areas, for which consolidated operational models do not exist. Psychological intervention in chronic disease, and specifically in MS, is certainly an area, up until now, explored by few, when one takes into consideration the global experience of illness of those affected, and not only one single aspect or psychopathological difficulty.

Putting the life of an ill person in the center

This project is based on a strong theoretical conception of development as a possibility of growth and adaptation that concerns the entire life cycle of the individual even in highly challenging critical situations of one's illness; in this development process, the individual plays an active and not merely reactive role.

As a consequence of this approach, the project aimed to place central aspects of people's lives: aspects that are of concern to any person, even those in good health, but with chronic illness gain particular relevance. It was not the intention to focus on sectoral aspects, however important, on the contrary, we want to address the underlying issues that concern the ability of the chronic patient, in our case the MS patient, to cope in a positive way of development and not regression, of adaptation and not of maladaptation to an existential condition of illness that will accompany one for the rest of their life. The more particular aspects have always been considered within a broader discussion; for example, symptom management has been examined in the context of promoting self-efficacy in the pursuit of meaningful personal goals, capable of giving meaning to one's life, consequently a life worth living.

In this perspective, the intervention takes into consideration the overall experience of a person in one's psychophysical unity, made up of body and psyche, in relationship with others. This means above all, considering the body, emotions and cognition, within their dynamic interactions. Consequently, activities are proposed, such as breathing and relaxation, which begin in the body on a path from "bottom to top", to better the psychic state while modifying the physiological state. At the same time, we work on modifying emotional states and managing stress through changing cognitive strategies for interpreting reality, in a path from "top to bottom", i.e., from the psyche to emotions and physiological states. Furthermore, interpersonal relations and good communication skills are taken into consideration, in particular with healthcare personnel and family members.

However, the intervention process is not limited only to these aspects, even given their grand importance; it focuses primarily and preliminary on identity and how to effectively pursue personal fulfillment and development that give meaning in one's life as a person with a chronic illness. It is therefore the existential aspects that are placed at the center of this intervention, in the belief that giving meaning to one's presence in the world is a fundamental need of every human being, even more pressing when life is profoundly upset by illness. These aspects are sometimes mistakenly considered beyond the scope of psychological intervention, in how philosophical or "spiritual"; on the contrary, they concern every human being and are at the center of this intervention project. In it, the use of strategies to promote self-efficacy is inserted within the research for new significant objectives with the capacity to give again a sense and purpose in one's life, making it worthwhile to live.

The non-psychopathological approach

In recent years, attention to the psychological aspects involved in living and managing MS has significantly increased. Despite this, psychological interventions for ill individuals are often based on both a theoretical and practical psychopathological approach. On the theoretical level, it is believed that disease "activates" a pre-existing psychopathological condition and therefore highlights significant difficulties of adaptation that were already inherent in the patient's personality. This is a direction that focuses neither on the great difficulties that a disease poses to the lives of individuals and development nor upon strengthening one's ability to cope with it. On a concrete level, with this approach, the psychologist is called into question, mostly upon recommendation of the neurologist, to cure the cases which it is believed that the ill person presents problems that make it difficult to treat the disease and relationships with healthcare personnel, i.e., non-compliant behavior, due to refusal of therapy. This also includes family relationships and working life, again conflictual or unmotivated abandonment of work. As a result, the person with MS who is referred to the psychologist implicitly experiences themselves as different from others. This increases the stigma toward those who "go to the psychologist" contributing to the distorted understanding of psychological intervention commonly thought of as for those who are crazy, maladjusted or at least strange. The poisoned fruit of this approach is the refusal, unfortunately still widespread, of psychological intervention viewed as stigmatizing. It is often accompanied by the claim of "wanting to do it alone with one's own determination or good will" without understanding that psychological help does not replace individual action but favors and strengthens it. The MS patient thus ends up being burdened not only with the already significant weight of the illness, but also having to cope with it alone.

This project was born from a very different theoretical and concrete approach. On a theoretical level, the emphasis is placed not on the person's latent pre-existing difficulties, but on its positive resources for effective adaptation in the process of personal development. These are resources that must be mobilized and supported to deal with an illness that poses extraordinary difficulties throughout one's life. It is therefore a question of prompting in the individual that which can favor effective active adaptation thus achieving personal development, also possible with illness. In this process, the individual plays a central role; the individual is the main actor of their development in the realities of everyday life, the relationship with one's life context, from family to one's broader social context. Not a psychopathological vision therefore, but a positive vision, which focuses on personal development and the active role played by the individual in the process of growth and adaptation. This is all clearly explained to the participants in the presentation of the intervention process: the problem is not the ill person, but the illness which poses enormous difficulties, representing a great and persistent challenge to personal development and well-being. Psychological support has the objective of providing tools to deal in the best possible way with the great and persistent difficulties posed by one's disease. Therefore, engaging in discussion with a psychologist does not represent a delegation or loss of autonomy but a way to elaborate and more quickly develop ways of adapting and behavioral strategies for continuing to live life with satisfaction. It certainly cannot be ruled out that rare pathological cases exist, but these are, in fact, limited cases, for which individual intervention continues to be foreseen and suggested.

On this basis, the general objective of psychological intervention is that individuals can live their lives to the fullest and continue to have personal development, thanks to effective adaptation within the limits posed by life with an illness: the emphasis is on life and not on illness. Personal development and better adaptation translate, in concrete terms, into greater well-being, less depression, greater optimism, greater quality of life, greater capacity to recognize and address negative emotions and promote positive ones, greater skills to communicate with family members and healthcare personnel. It must be reiterated that all of this is also reflected directly and indirectly on the physical level, due to the psychophysical unity of the individual. Personal development and effective adaptation not only make one live better, but allow you to achieve better therapeutic results and create a cooperative relationship between patient and one's care staff. A positive therapeutic relationship, capable of coping with many difficulties and numerous critical moments, is in fact decisive in the treatment of a chronic degenerative disease such as MS.

Group intervention

The proposed intervention is not individual but group-based (see Chapter 3). This choice is time-saving, and therefore money, but above all, it is motivated by the advantages that the participants derive from the comparison with other people who find themselves in the same condition as newly diagnosed and experience the same period of life cycle (youth, adulthood and mature age). The participants consequently share the same developmental tasks and find themselves facing similar life situations: for example, for young people, the conquest of emotional and economic autonomy from their family of origin, entry into working life, the construction of lasting emotional relationships. This similarity promotes mutual understanding and allows individuals to benefit from the experience of others. Comparison with the other members of the group also encourages everyone's involvement, both because it facilitates the sense of belonging ("we are a group and we help each other") and because it stimulates introspection, in-depth analysis and individual creativity. For example, a member may suggest a strategy they use to manage a symptom to other participants in new ways, different from the usual ones or even ones never thought of, to manage the same symptom or similar symptoms.

An intervention and research project

The close relationship between intervention and research: The initial phase of evaluating intervention

Among the main characteristics of this project is the juxtaposition between intervention and research, with positive repercussions for both, as demonstrated by the numerous scientific publications (see Appendix 6): this relationship constitutes one of the most important strong points of this project (see Chapter 4). For this purpose, the working team was made up of people with skills and experience in both the clinical and research fields, they are the scientific manager and creator of the project, a psychologist with the task of leading the intervention groups, a psychologist with research tasks, and a psychologist with research tasks and joint participation in some intervention activities. The members of the team coordinate with the promoting entities, within their sphere of competence, for the implementation of interventions and research.

Before being proposed fully, the project was first of all preliminarily evaluated, in terms of its feasibility and effectiveness, through the comparison between an intervention group and a comparison group that participated in information meetings on topics of interest to those suffering from MS (for example, nutrition). In this first phase, the participants of the intervention group were not only newly diagnosed and there were four meetings, followed by a meeting after six months and another after a year (see Chapter 4, paragraph *The project for newly diagnosed patients*). Conducting comparison research in the psychological field involves far greater difficulties than a classic therapeutic trial, such as, to verify the validity of a drug. In fact, we are dealing with real people, with all the variety and complexity of the life that they continue to live. Therefore, rigorous isolation of the variables is not possible. This is why conducting research in the psychological field with concrete individualities, not in an experimental situation, is more complex. However, this does not mean that it is impossible. We believe that our project, as it was carried out, demonstrates that it is possible to conduct quality research, with a strong theoretical framework and valid tools, achieves communicable and comparable results, even in real-life conditions. In this regard, I want to underscore that attention to the persons, to their well-being, to the usefulness of the experience for each of the participants, was and is always our first thought. For example, if asking certain questions in the questionnaire could risk causing discomfort, we decided to ignore it; if final questionnaire, with the addition of other useful and interesting scales, ended up being too long (fatigue, let's not forget, is among the most relevant symptoms of MS), we decided to find other solutions. The amount of time and the questions themselves were functional first and foremost for the well-being of the participants, not for the research itself at all costs.

This initial phase confirmed the validity of the project. In addition to the very high level of participation in the groups (minimal withdrawals), the participants unanimously assessed their group experience as positive (topics addressed, management, materials provided, place where the meetings were held) in the assessment questionnaire (*My point of view*) and in the focus groups.

The audio recording of the meetings highlighted that participation in the group was experienced as positive, fostering change.

In addition to the subjective evaluations, the results of the intervention participants were compared with those of the comparison group in their responses to the different scales of the *Me and my life* questionnaire; the participants in the intervention obtained better results than those in the comparison group on the various scales that measured the variables on which the intervention was carried out (such as well-being, depression, quality of life).

Adding to this analysis is the collegial evaluation by the working team, which concerned the progress of both the individual groups during their various meetings and of the project in general. This evaluation allowed some improvements to be made to the intervention project, proposed to the newly diagnosed patients. The changes did not concern the topics covered and the general methodology, but only the guiding outline, in order to take into account the different temporal experience of the participants' illness. Furthermore, the meetings from four were increased to five, as the number was insufficient.

Evaluation over the years

The verification of the results has continued over the years and has made use of various tools (see Chapter 4).

An observer was always present in the meetings, with the task of recording, on the basis of an observation grid (Appendix 3), what happened in the group in relation to the contents, management, and participants. These observations provided important material for the "process" evaluation by the working team, with respect to both a single group and several groups and intervention in general. It should be underscored that the people involved have always participated in the scheduled and ongoing meetings of the working team: from those who were mostly dedicated to in-depth research to those who had the task of leading the intervention groups.

Already in the initial phase, for the subjective evaluation of the group experience, the aforementioned *My point of view* questionnaire was used, administered at the end of the fifth meeting, to which the participants' judgments were added in the focus group (carried out one year after the end of the meetings) regarding the topics covered, the management, the material provided and the location of the meetings. Over the years, there have been very few participant withdrawals.

The *Me and my life* questionnaire was instead administered at the beginning of the first meeting, at the end of the fifth, after six months and after a year, thus allowing the results of the intervention to be evaluated not only immediately but also in the long term, with a longitudinal research plan. For comparison, the questionnaire was administered over time to newly diagnosed people who were not participating in the intervention. The questionnaire has been expanded over the years and groups together different scales, selected in relation to the aspects covered and the objectives of the intervention (see Chapter 4, paragraph *The project for newly diagnosed patients*).

The results of the questionnaires have allowed us to delve deeper into some topics of great psychological relevance over time, to create a new tool for assessing self-efficacy, and to test hypotheses of relationships between variables (see Chapter 4). These are important theoretical results for the knowledge of the psychological problems of people suffering from MS that continue to lack today, theoretical results that give further indications for intervention.

Collaboration between different entities

The project is the result of formalized and continuous collaboration between different public and private bodies none of which, alone, could have supported the weight of such an intertwined and complex activity, for such a long period of time. Coordinating intervention and research in a lasting way, over the years, requires patience and a spirit of collaboration on the part of those who work in the various bodies involved: as we have already underlined, bodies are first and foremost people and not simple acronyms. Only in this way, can the inevitable problems and moments of difficulty be overcome, with results that amply repay the efforts made, avoiding the risk of impromptu and ephemeral initiatives, however interesting.

This collaboration made it possible to conduct the meetings of the intervention groups in places other than hospital or outpatient clinics, inevitably associated with lived experiences often in a negative way, such as therapies or hospitalizations. Thanks to the Cosso Foundation, we are able to have a place of extraordinary beauty (the Miradolo Castle, surrounded by a large park) normally open to the public for naturalistic and cultural activities, in particular exhibitions. This location has been particularly appreciated by the participants over the years, despite the fact that it posed greater organizational problems, being a decentralized location. The beauty of the place and its regular use for other activities have contributed to transmitting a positive message of valorization and at the same time of normality.

In Box 1.2, we present a summary of the project.

Box 1.2   Summary of the project

The psychological intervention group project for people who have recently received the diagnosis of MS was born in 2009 from the fruitful meeting between science and personal experience and from the collaboration between different entities. It is a dynamic project, structured over time and open to modifications, in the continuous mutual relationship between intervention and research, between experience and its evaluation.

Goals

The general objective of the psychological intervention group project is to *encourage personal development and effective adaptation*, so that people with MS can live their lives to the fullest and with satisfaction even within the limits set by the disease. The specific objectives are greater quality of life, greater well-being, less depression, greater optimism, more adaptive coping strategies, greater ability to cope with negative emotions and promote positive ones, greater ability to communicate with family members and healthcare personnel.

Methodology

The intervention is carried out with group meetings led by a psychologist; in them, the discussion between the participants allows for exchanges and in-depth analysis, while the presence of the facilitator guarantees collaboration and focus on the chosen themes. There are five meetings, on an every two-week basis, followed by a recall meeting (follow-up) after six months and another to recall and evaluate the experience after a year (focus group).

Phases of the project

The first two years (2009–2011) had the aim of evaluating the validity of the project and the proposed activities, through the comparison between an intervention group (with four meetings) and a comparison group. The recipients were, in this phase, people with MS even many years after diagnosis. The groups were organized based on age, identifying three groups: young people, adults and mature people. Based on the positive results obtained, it was decided to continue the activity, dedicating it specifically to newly diagnosed people, with some modifications. Since the number of meetings proved insufficient, they went from four to five, again every two weeks, followed by a recall meeting after six months (follow-up) and another to recall and evaluate the experience after a year (focus group).

The group interventions were carried out continuously, from 2011 to to-day, in the spring and autumn periods, always grouping people by age group.

Meeting place

The meetings always take place on the Castle premises of Miradolo (S. Secondo di Pinerolo, Turin) made available by the Cosso Foundation.

Recipients

Recipients are the people who received from less than three years their di-agnoses of MS and who have a mild to medium level of disability (EDSS up to 5.5).

Activity

The meetings consider crucial aspects for the development of the person in their *daily life with the illness*: identity, the search for meaning, the effec-tive realization of significant objectives. Alongside these, other aspects are examined that can favor or make such personal development difficult: stress management, effective management of symptoms, emotions, relationships between thoughts and emotions and communication. Relaxation exercises are also proposed.

The participants are asked to do "homework" with the help of specific materials, to be done between one meeting and another, to delve deeper into the proposed themes on a personal level.

Assessment

To evaluate the results, the following different tools are used:

- Compilation of an observation form by an observer (in the first two years: audio recording of the meetings).
- Process evaluation by the working team.
- The experience evaluation questionnaire (*My point of view*), administered to participants at the end of the five meetings.
- The focus group after one year.
- The *Me and my life* questionnaire, administered to participants at the beginning of the first meeting, at the end of the fifth, after six months and after an year. The questionnaire, expanded over the years, groups together various scales, in relation to the objectives. For comparison, this questionnaire was administered to newly diagnosed people who were not participating in the intervention.

Results

The specific objectives of the intervention were achieved. In addition, some topics of psychological relevance were explored in depth; a new self-efficacy assessment tool was created and hypotheses regarding the relationship between variables relevant to the well-being and better adaptation of people with MS were tested.

The recipients of the intervention

The newly diagnosed people

The recipients of the project presented here are newly diagnosed MS patients, i.e., people within the first three years of receiving the diagnosis. This period is in fact identified by the literature (Dennison et al., 2009; Kern et al., 2009), confirming our clinical experience, as particularly critical. For the person, it involves facing the diagnosis of a chronic neurodegenerative disease for which there are no definitive treatments today and which is immediately associated in the collective imagination with serious motor disability: in simple words, with the wheelchair. This identification is erroneous, both due to the great variety of consequences of MS on the functioning of the body, not all of which are visible from the outside, and due to recent therapies, which allow for a more favorable impact on the long-term trend of the disease. Despite this, the imagery defined by the wheelchair continues to be the prevalent one.

In the period following one's diagnosis, the person experiences strong negative emotions, ranging from denial to anger, from fear to depression (Giordano et al., 2011; Janssen et al., 2003; Possa et al., 2017). Even though it is the moment in which psychological support is most necessary, newly diagnosed people often refuse it, overwhelmed by anguish for the future and the difficulty of dealing with their own strong emotional experiences. Isolation and closing up within oneself are frequently critical consequences. For this reason, it is essential that the psychological support intervention is offered to everyone, as a normal therapeutic proposal that integrates the pharmacological one. And it is essential that it is offered immediately, at the most critical moment, helping the person to not aggravate their suffering and begin to cope with the illness as best as possible right from the start. Considering the disease lasts a lifetime and progresses, at least in the first few years, mostly alternating phases between remission and worsening. Psychological intervention after the diagnosis does not in itself guarantee that the ill person will not experience other critical moments in their future. However, it allows us to set up positive ways of dealing with an illness that will last one's entire existence, by starting on a path that looks to the future and the possibilities of personal fulfillment, without remaining entangled in negative feelings and regret for what the illness has taken away.

Acceptance of the disease thus becomes concretely possible, as the result of a successful adaptation to the new condition and its evolution over time (see Chapter 2); adaptation that is achieved, in concrete terms, thanks to the active reorganization

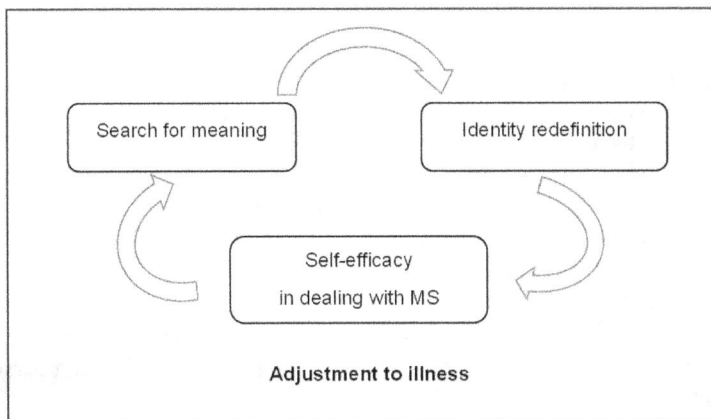

Figure 1.1 Diagram of the circular relationship between the intervention aspects covered.

of oneself and one's identity and the identification of significant objectives that the person knows how to achieve. At the same time, the lower emotional activation resulting from acceptance and good adaptation allows the ill person to be in a virtuous circle, to dedicate oneself more to these tasks. We deliberately chose to not directly propose the topic of illness acceptance in the groups, the risk being too theoretical and abstract, without being able to concretely promote positive prospects for personal fulfillment. We prefer to bring out this important aspect indirectly, almost without naming it, as the result of a good adaptation (see Figure 1.1).

The project is also applicable to people for whom several years have passed since the diagnosis, and it has in fact been applied in the evaluation phase. Considering the intertwining of the evolution of the illness with the changes that concern the different moments of life requires a continuous review of the significant goals, capable of concretizing the identity, and of the strategies to achieve them.

The level of disability

For participation in the groups, a mild and medium level of disability was chosen, with an EDSS of up to 5.5 (see Box 1.1). This choice is not motivated only by the fact that people who have recently been diagnosed generally have a low level of disability, included in this range, but it is coherently connected to the objectives and characteristics of the project themselves. These concern people who, due to their level of disability, are still involved in working or family life, and must be helped to find new ways to maintain this vital commitment, even if in a different or reduced way. For this reason, even the first evaluation phase of the project was always aimed at people with a mild or medium level of disability.

It should also be considered that the condition of having a certain diagnosis of MS, but with a low degree of disability, is more frequent today than in the past. In fact, greater diagnostic accuracy, thanks above all to nuclear MRI, has led in recent years to diagnosing MS earlier even in people, both young and old, who present ambiguous or not very evident symptoms. This is undoubtedly an advantage, because it saves the person a long and tiring diagnostic process and allows timely pharmacological intervention. On a psychological level, however, there may be greater resistance and less awareness of the disease, to the point of its denial. On a social level, the reduced visibility of the patient can lead to an erroneous evaluation of one's condition by others, making it difficult to recognize the needs of the ill person. At the same time, advances in therapies now allow many people with MS to continue to lead (however, with challenges) an apparently normal working and family life for years. As a result, the person with MS is today increasingly "the person next door" and can no longer be identified solely with the severely disabled.

Despite this, the group psychological intervention project also provides guidance for people with a higher level of disability. In fact, the disabled person has the psychological need to still give meaning to their life and to realize their identity through significant activities, achieved effectively despite the serious limits imposed by the disease; at the same time, one needs to learn to manage symptoms and emotions, to cope with stress and to communicate effectively. The themes addressed in the group psychological intervention process therefore remain valid. However, in this case, the presentation of these topics and the concrete activities proposed will need to be substantially revised and restructured.

The same can be said for other chronic pathologies, currently on the increase in the Western world, such as diabetes and cardiovascular diseases. Also in this case, the project can provide useful indications in its theoretical bases and basic objectives, while the proposed activities must be re-calibrated in relation to the specificities of the different pathologies (Bonino et al., 2025).

References

Bonino, S. (2021). *Coping with chronic illness. Theories, issues and lived experiences.* Routledge.

Bonino, S., Calandri, E., Cattelino, E. (2025). Living with a chronic illness as a challenge to psychological development: The role of personal identity, sense of coherence and perceived self-efficacy, Social Sciences & Humanities Open, 11,101620.

Dennison, L., Moss-Morris, R., & Chalder, T. (2009). A review of psychological correlates of adjustment in patients with multiple sclerosis. *Clinical Psychology Review, 29*, 141–153.

Giordano, A., Granella, F., Lugaresi, A., Martinelli, V., Trojano, M., Confalonieri, P., Radice, D., & Solari, A. (2011). Anxiety and depression in multiple sclerosis patients around diagnosis. *Journal of Neurological Sciences, 307*, 86–91.

Janssen, A. C. J. W., van Doorn, P. A., de Boer, J. B., van der Meche´, F. G. A., Passchier, J., & Hintzen, R. Q. (2003). Impact of recently diagnosed multiple sclerosis on quality of life, anxiety, depression, and distress of patients and partners. *Acta Neurologica Scandinavica, 108*, 389–395.

Kern, S., Schrempf, W., Schneider, H., Schultheiss, T., Reichmann, H., & Ziemssen, T. (2009). Neurological disability, psychological distress, and health-related quality of life in MS patients within the first three years after diagnosis. *Multiple Sclerosis, 15*, 752–758.

Kurtzke, J. F. (1983). Rating neurologic impairment in multiple sclerosis: An Expanded Disability Status Scale (EDSS). *Neurology, 33*, 1444–1452.

Possa, M. F., Minacapelli, E., Canale, S., Comi, G., Martinelli, V., & Falautano, M. (2017). The first year after diagnosis: Psychological impact on people with multiple sclerosis. *Psychology, Health and Medicine, 22*, 1063–1071.

2 The theoretical foundations

*Emanuela Calandri, Martina Borghi
and Federica Graziano*

Multiple sclerosis (MS) as a challenge to development in the life cycle (Emanuela Calandri)

As mentioned in the previous chapter, the research and intervention project is characterized by having solid theoretical foundations, with specific origins in developmental psychology and health psychology. This chapter will illustrate the theoretical concepts underlying the project to understand how they are applied to the practice of intervention.

Starting from a perspective now widely widespread in developmental psychology studies, let us first define what is meant by "development over the life cycle". Development is defined as incremental change, that is, change that leads to greater complexity, coherence, and stability in a person and their relationships with the environment (Ford & Lerner, 1992). According to the life cycle perspective, development is a lifelong process of change. Changes over one's life cycle are traditionally distinguished into normative and non-normative changes (Baltes, 1997; Hendry & Kloep, 2002). Some regulatory changes are common to all people: for example, changes related to biological factors, such as puberty. Other normative changes are of a social nature, common to many people and are age-related, as well as being regulated by laws (for example, entering compulsory schooling, reaching legal age). Other regulatory changes are expected with respect to a specific individual evolutionary moment, even if they are not regulated by written rules and change in relation to different social and cultural contexts (for example entry into the world of work). Non-normative changes are experienced by a limited number of people; these are events that occur out of phase with respect to the "developmental tasks" of a certain age (for example, a pregnancy in adolescence), or events linked to particular historical circumstances (i.e., political conflicts or war) or even specific events that affect the individual, such as an accident or illness. From a developmental psychology perspective, every situation of change during the individual life cycle represents a moment of crisis that requires the individual to undergo an adaptation process. However, while regulatory changes are expected and predictable and generally represent less challenging situations for an individual, non-normative changes present more taxing challenges. The ability to adaptively

DOI: 10.4324/9781003484400-2

address these challenges can in turn translate into an opportunity for growth and development (Hendry & Kloep, 2002).

The need to adapt to one's disease, understood as a non-normative change in the life cycle, arises both in cases of acute pathologies, usually delimited in time and followed by recovery, even over a considerably long period of time. Above all, in the case of chronic illness, such as MS, which is by definition non-curable and tends to worsen over time. The challenge for the individual consists, in particular, living the experience of chronic illness within the trajectory of individual development, through an adaptation process that is not a passive acceptance of the condition of suffering, but engaging in an active and continuous search for a new equilibrium.

MS is diagnosed predominantly in young adulthood, between the ages of twenty and thirty, a period of life in which individuals must face various developmental tasks, including making choices regarding study and future, working careers, achieving an economic independence from their family of origin, establishing an equal relationship with one's parents, engaging in an intimate emotional relationship and making choices about becoming a parent (Arnett, 2000; Sharon, 2015).

The diagnosis of an illness in young adulthood appears as a moment of profound discontinuity in one's individual life cycle, as a real and specific biographical fracture. A young person finds themselves having to face the double challenge of becoming an adult and recognizing oneself as ill. The topic of pediatric MS will not be addressed here, as it is not in the scope of this work, even if increasing levels early diagnoses forcefully prompt the need to consider the challenges posed by chronic disease to an adolescent.

MS on the other hand can also be diagnosed in full adulthood (between thirty and fifty years of age) or even at a more advanced age, often in individuals who have already had a long history of the pathology, not diagnosed in the past as MS due to diagnostic tools that were less accurate than current ones. At whatever age one is diagnosed, the disease always represents a challenge that imposes the need for a profound redefinition of oneself in relation to their developmental life cycle tasks. For example, in adulthood it imposes the need to redefine already consolidated roles at work, attaining early retirement, or even to reconcile the difficulties of managing symptoms and therapies with the fulfillment of parental duties.

At any age, MS therefore represents a profound and dramatic transformation to be faced, by appealing to individual and contextual resources, in constructing a new and continuous process of adaptation. In this regard, the perspective of developmental psychology reminds us that the individual plays a fundamental role through the actions one exerts on reality (Magnusson & Stattin, 2006). Therefore, the individual is the protagonist of their own development, in a bidirectional and continuous process of influence between the individual themself given one's limits and potential, within the context of one's constraints and resources. Being protagonists of one's own development in chronic illness therefore implies actively seeking an adaptation to the illness, with the awareness that it will not be achieved once and for all, but is a slow process, lasting through time, with moments of crisis and subsequent readjustments, in relationship to the course of the disease and individual changes (Bonino, 2021).

In the following paragraphs, the psychological aspects on which this intervention model is based will be addressed from a theoretical point of view. First, we will examine the constructs of personal identity, sense of coherence and perceived self-efficacy. As mentioned in the previous chapter, these are three crucial aspects for the development of a person that are austerely tested by the diagnosis of an illness. But, at the same time, they represent an individual's resources on which one can work to encourage development and adaptation. Since the disease has a strong impact, through its numerous symptoms, on the functioning of the body and consequently also on the psychological aspects just indicated, we will subsequently consider the symptoms of the disease and their consequences on emotional experiences and on self-representation. Finally, some aspects that can promote individual development will be covered, such as the management of negative emotions, the relationship between emotions and thoughts and effective communication.

Identity, sense of coherence and perceived self-efficacy (Emanuela Calandri)

"Who am I?" Redefining one's identity with the disease

Identity is defined as the sense of continuity and unity that everyone experiences throughout their lives, despite continuous physical, psychological and social changes (Bosma & Kunnen, 2001). Transition periods in the life cycle generally represent moments in which a redefinition of one's identity is required: a split situation that requires restructuring one's identity, generally persons manage this process with success. The diagnosis of a chronic disease, such as MS, on the contrary represents a threat and a profound fracture in the individual's sense of identity (Breakwell, 1983; Charmaz, 1983). In fact, it suddenly and lastingly changes the functioning of the body and the self-image, as well as projects, the possibilities of realization and the consequent social roles in which the individual is engaged (Weinreich & Saunderson, 2003).

The identity fracture is particularly evident for young adults. They are in fact in a period of the life cycle in which they explore different prospects in the fields of study, work and relationships toward a progressive definition of an adult identity (Arnett, 2000). The diagnosis at this age presents itself as a profound rupture in their planning. The individual suddenly perceives themselves as ill and, as mentioned above, must face the double challenge of redefining one's identity as a young adult and as a person suffering from a chronic illness. However, even at other ages the diagnosis represents a splintering between before and after. An individual in full adulthood will most likely have already defined their identity in their work and family context, but one's role in the different contexts will necessarily have to be redefined, in relation to the difficulties posed by one's disease. For example, requiring changes in the work context, or the need for help in managing parenting tasks, in more serious cases the individual may end up losing their working and social role, consequently a profound restructuring of the oneself is necessary, discernibly in relation to the limits and possibilities granted by the disease.

Redefining one's identity following the diagnosis means reorganizing one's future perspective and goals, taking into account limitations and disabilities related to the disease, but also possibilities and resources to advance a new self-image that includes the disease, but is not absorbed by it. Identity restructuring is not a given once and for all, but must be a continuous process through time, in relation to the fluctuating and unpredictable progress of one's illness.

The few studies in the international literature on the relationship between identity and MS highlight how the ability to redefine one's identity with their illness is linked to fewer depressive symptoms and a higher quality of life and greater psychological well-being (Irvine et al., 2009; Tabuteau-Harrison et al., 2016). Redefining life goals with the disease and integrating the disease into individual identity therefore represent central processes capable of promoting psychological well-being.[1]

"What gives meaning to my life?" Building a sense of coherence with illness

Individual identity materializes in significant actions, in objectives that give meaning to life and make it worth living. The need to find meaning in one's existence is characteristic of all human beings throughout the life cycle (Frankl, 1946, 2011). Moments of transition and turning point make this need stronger, particularly if they involve non-normative changes. Specifically, the disease represents a moment of transition that brings with it a situation of unknown, of incomprehensibility, where nothing seems to make sense anymore. Questioning oneself about the meaning of one's life therefore becomes fundamental to starting and continuing the process of adaptation to one's illness over time. A person suffering from MS can in fact perceive that their life has meaning when they create significant goals to engage in, despite the constraints of the illness (Bonino, 2021).

The construct of "sense of coherence" developed by Antonovsky (1987) refers to the way in which the person perceives, interprets and tries to make sense of the stimuli that come from both the internal and external world. More specifically, the sense of coherence represents the individual's ability to respond to stressful situations through the ability to understand what is happening (comprehensibility), the perception of having resources to cope with the situation (manageability) and the ability to make sense of the situation one is experiencing (meaningfulness). MS is an illness with an unpredictable course of unknown origin and without definitive treatments, profoundly influencing the individual's sense of coherence. Faced with the uncertainty and unpredictability of this illness, personal goals and the possibilities of their realization are called into question, with the risk of disengagement and absence of investment. The construction of meaning is linked to a positive adaptation to the conditions of chronic illness (Eriksson & Lindstrom, 2006) and to MS in particular (Pakenham, 2007). This takes on the form of accepting the challenges posed by one's illness, in the search for new objectives that can be addressed and that are realistically within one's reach, in the commitment to achieving new goals deemed personally significant and worthy of investment, therefore capable of giving a feeling of fulfillment and personal value, recovering the possibilities for action and planning (Bonino, 2021). The search for meaning concerns both the initial phases of the illness, following the diagnosis, which represents a moment of profound break with the past, and the following periods, in a continuous adaptation to the relapses and remissions of the illness, which each time bring with them the need to redefine your life goals.

"What am I capable of doing?" Promote self-efficacy in disease management

The possibility of redefining one's identity and finding meaning in one's experience of life with the illness can only become reality if the individual perceives they have the necessary skills to face this task. It is for this reason, the third psychological construct on which the theoretical model of our intervention is based, represented by perceived self-efficacy, that is the belief in one's ability to implement the actions necessary to obtain the desired results (Bandura, 1997). The individual must perceive they are capable of achieving the objectives that are significant to them, giving meaning to one's life in pursuit of their identity with illness.

The symptoms and difficulties of MS profoundly undermine the individual's feeling of self-efficacy. People perceive that they are no longer able to do what they used to do in their work, family and social spheres, compounded by experiencing failures that further reduce their sense of effectiveness. On the other hand, defenses such as denial of difficulties and overestimation of one's abilities also lead to failure and a lower sense of self-efficacy. It then becomes important to maintain a good level of self-efficacy starting from the recognition of one's limits and resources available.

Promoting self-efficacy has been shown to be useful in managing chronic disease (Aujoulat, 2007; Holman & Lorig, 2004), particularly in promoting behavioral changes (Bandura, 1997). Studies in the literature highlight how, even in the case of MS, greater self-efficacy in managing one's illness is linked not only to greater adherence to therapies (Fraser et al., 2001) and greater physical activity (Ferrier et al., 2010), but also has broader positive effects on psychological adaptation and quality of life (Dennison et al., 2009; Schmitt et al., 2014; Wilski & Tasiemski, 2016). The literature therefore suggests the importance of intervening on strengthening self-efficacy, evaluating individual abilities and limits, identifying significant and achievable objectives and implementing adequate strategies and the necessary action plans. As already said regarding the construct of identity and the search for meaning, this work on the feeling of personal self-efficacy must be continuous over time, not just once and for all, renewed on the occasion not only of large, but also of small variations linked to the progression of one's illness.

Symptoms and emotional experiences (Martina Borghi)

Symptoms and perception of the body

A person is a psychophysical unit, as developments in scientific knowledge increasingly underscore (Bottaccioli & Bottaccioli, 2020; Porges, 2011). On the one hand, changes in the body caused by MS have significant consequences on a psychological level, on the other they are continually gauged and interpreted by the person who suffers them. Hence, during the life journey with illness the perception of one's body, its characteristics, its limits and its residual potential can change profoundly.

A meta-synthesis of 292 qualitative research studies conducted by Paterson (2001) shows how living with a chronic illness can be understood as a continuous and constantly evolving process. The author derived from this analysis the model of "shifting perspectives" (shifting perspectives model), which provides an explanation of the varied regard people with chronic illness give symptoms over time, which can sometimes be exaggerated or even harmful to one's health.

Phenomenological studies of MS that have focused on the period from diagnosis to the first years of life with illness reveal a profound sense of bodily alienation (De Ceuninck van Capelle et al., 2016; Edwards et al., 2008; Finlay, 2003). A review of studies on body image in people with MS (Di Cara et al., 2019) highlighted that, due to afflictions experienced in the present and presumed future impairments, the person modifies their mental image of their body from the beginning of the illness.

Toombs (1992) states that part of the uncertainty experienced in degenerative diseases relates to the fact that one must learn and relearn how to negotiate the relationship between one's body and the surrounding world on an ongoing basis. The thought "I can do it again" can no longer be taken for granted.

A recent study (Stevens et al., 2019) examined the level of body image dissatisfaction (BID) in a sample of 151 people with MS. Although these generally show the same levels of satisfaction as the general population, some variables predict higher scores of dissatisfaction; in particular, women with a higher body mass index and more severe depressive symptoms report high scores on the stigma scale, which measures the perceived frequency of negative reactions from others toward them, linked to the disease (for example: "Because of the my illness some people avoid me").

Given the evidence in the literature on the negative effects of body dissatisfaction, health behaviors and mood, it would be important to explore whether other factors influence BID in people with MS. For example, it would be interesting to explore the correlation between dissatisfaction with one's body image, and the weakening of walking or other symptoms.

A qualitative study conducted in the Netherlands (van der Meide et al., 2018) highlights how the bodily experience of people with MS can reflect a continuous oscillation between four experiential dimensions that follow one another over time and which correspond to adaptive responses to one's ill body: "bodily uncertainty, having a precious body, being a different body, mindful body". The individual then passes through different phases and oscillates in a process that alternates between bodily hypervigilance, with self-observation interpreting every change as a sign of illness and worsening, to a progressive attention to the body not necessarily understood as an uncomfortable shell. It therefore becomes clear how important it is to encourage the process of acquiring greater body awareness and a perception of the body as an internal resource from which to draw stability and security. Consequently, consciously focusing attention on the body can serve to cultivate a sense of well-being, whereby the negative effects of MS only temporarily dominate the experience. Urging the modification of defense mechanisms that aim at bodily disappearance such as denial, displacement and dissociation, to the idea of the body as support, is a central practice in psychological support.

The construction of body image is inextricably linked to identity, self-esteem, appearing, sexual function and social relationships, and therefore, body image and psychological aspects are closely interconnected. The body is a fundamental part of the construction of one's identity.

Despite the very wide range of symptoms that can affect people with MS, some of them occur more frequently. Furthermore, each symptom can change over time both in the intensity in which it manifests itself and in its duration. The symptoms most complained about by people are fatigue, mood disorders, balance and walking difficulties, vision disorders, sensitivity disorders and strength deficits, bladder problems, and finally cognitive disorders.

Each symptom alters the perception of one's body, and for this reason, intervening early by reeducating to listen to the body, understanding it not only as a repository of unpleasant and disabling perceptions, is essential.

Below (Box 2.1) are some symptoms and examples of the descriptions that patients most often use to explain what they perceive on a bodily level.[2]

Box 2.1   Symptoms as perceived by the patient

Symptoms	*Patient descriptions*
Hyperesthesia = pain; burning	Being a human torch (burning); feeling pinched by a simple caress; feeling pain in the body part that has just been touched by something or someone
Paresthesia = tingling	Pins; ants; needles, itching
Hypoesthesia = decreased tactile sensibility/thermal/pain	Numb or weak limb (sometimes dead); do not perceive contact with objects, people; bandaging sensation; do not feel hot or cold; do not feel pain after burns
Dysesthesia = abnormal based sensations	Elephant leg; wooden leg
Anesthesia = total loss of sensation	Dead limb
Trigeminal neuralgia	Electric shocks in one part of the face, such as at the corner of the nose or mouth; feeling of torn skin
Diplopia = double vision	foggy, blurry vision
Optic neuritis = decreased monocular vision + pain	Black spots; not seeing a part of space; blurred vision; pangs behind the eye
Fatigue	Continuous or sudden tiredness that is difficult to manage and tolerate; head muffled; mushy brain; confused perceptions

---

Sensitivity disorders and pain

Sometimes, one's bodily perception is *amplified* by a symptom, as in the case of hyperesthesia, manifesting itself in pain, burning or stinging sensations. Other times, the perception is *altered,* as in the case of paresthesia, presenting itself in the form of tingling – often described as needles or pins in the limbs or other parts of the body – or in the form of sensations in the absence of a stimulus, such as being touched by a thread or a veil. In other cases, perception is reduced due to hypoesthesia, which presents itself as numbness, up to the total absence of sensitivity, in which case the body is anesthetized in some points.

Sensitivity disorders contribute in particular to altering the body map and the perception of one's boundaries. It may happen, for example, that it is no longer clear where one's body ends and where an external object begins, so it is necessary to ascertain with the help of sight whether the object grasped with the hands, held in the lap or lifted, is really firm between the limbs. Sometimes, people report having completely lost sensitivity when instead there is an alteration that has changed tactile sensibility; consequently, a more incisive touch and stronger pressure is needed to be able to feel. Acquiring greater awareness about hyposensitivity is very important in order to remodulate one's tactile relationship with the world and recover this fundamental bodily resource which has not disappeared but is modified.

On the contrary, in case of hypersensitivity one's touch turns into a painful stimulus because the person feels electric shocks, or a burning sensation, even if something has barely touched the parts of the body where this symptom is most present (allodynia). Hyperalgesia can also occur independently of a tactile stimulus, whereby the person perceives pain as a constant or intermittent presence that affects different parts of the body. More often, "belt" pain, a feeling of tightness between the lower part of the chest and the waist, is described as wearing a belt that is too tight. In whatever form it occurs, pain is a common symptom that is estimated to affect more than 75% of people (Solaro et al., 2013).

Pain can be present at any time during the course of the illness, and patients can experience pain in different parts of the body at the same time. Furthermore, pain may be secondary to other symptoms, such as spasticity, fatigue, and mood disorders (Solaro et al., 2013).

Of all these invisible symptoms, tingling is the most often reported. If at first glance paresthesias may seem less disabling than other symptoms, in reality this constant annoyance can greatly wear down the tolerance of those who experience it. In fact, especially when its presence is continuous, it is difficult to be able to rest effectively or concentrate on what you are doing, because one's attention is seized by the unpleasant sensation of having needles pricking your skin (Tihanyi et al., 2018). Especially at the beginning of the disease process, when adaptation to this symptom has not yet occurred, it is not unusual to hear people talk about their body as a cumbersome and painful shell that elicits emotions such as anger and frustration.

People express negative thoughts by saying things like: "If I could, I'd take my arm off", or "I hate this part of my body". Over time, the attack aimed at the body can be replaced by a strategy of indifference toward it, and therefore toward one's own physical sensations and emotions, or by a disidentification, as if the body that perceives those stimuli was not one's own. These strategies may seem adaptive at first, because the person tends to feel less sore, tingling or with altered sensation. However, it is necessary to replace these modes of disconnection with more adaptive ones, to avoid a gradual dissociation from one's body and instead facilitate a reconnection to one's bodily self.

Fatigue

Fatigue, which is the most frequent symptom and in many respects the most complicated to deal with (Gullvi et al., 2003; Miller & Soundy, 2017), also contributes to body dysperception. Daily actions such as showering, dressing, preparing meals are undermined by the presence of fatigue described as *continuous* or, more rarely, *sudden*. The body is invaded by a weakness that prevents or hinders carrying out actions. For example, women may have difficulty putting on makeup because their arms have to remain raised and they feel like they don't have enough strength, while for men it can be tiring to shave. Washing your hair becomes even worse, because rubbing the shampoo, putting pressure on the scalp and moving your arms and hands becomes a difficult and wearisome movement. As a result, drying your hair with your arms raised and supporting the weight of the hairdryer can be truly exhausting. When the symptom of fatigue can become overwhelming, beginning with one of the first morning actions of the day, i.e., pulling aside the covers to get out of bed can be grueling.

Fatigue may be associated with tremor because the muscles are making a high effort. This secondary symptom can create difficulty with fine movements, such as putting on eye makeup, buttoning a shirt or putting on earrings. It is therefore clear that, especially in cases of overwhelming fatigue, taking care of your body is a commitment that can become exasperating.

In cases where a person is able to accept and rework these struggles in constructive terms, one uses their own resources in seeking effective compliance to fit their new situation. Sometimes, tailoring to one's situation in an accommodating way means changing your hairstyle (for example, keeping your hair shorter or your beard longer) or favoring clothes without or with fewer buttonholes to button. Revamping your clothing and image in this way does not necessarily mean completely renouncing how you were before MS and fatigue were present. It is a process that certainly begins with abandoning some previous habits and ways of taking care of oneself, but replacing them with others that are equally significant and satisfying. Other times, however, change is a process to which the individual is forced by circumstances, but remains unaccepted on an emotional level; consequently, the component of renouncing how one was before illness is the only relevant aspect for the person.

Fatigue is a particularly subtle symptom because it is part of the symptoms called "invisible", i.e., it represents a subjective state that is not externally visible to the observer. This characteristic can create incorrect interpretations of the behavior of the person with MS, who may be judged as not very strong-willed, not very motivated or lazy. In fact, fatigue is often underestimated or, even worse, not taken into consideration or incorrectly gauged by those near the patient. This causes obvious emotional discomfort for those who have to live with fatigue, often prompting misunderstandings in relationships with others, who express value judgments without realizing that it does not depend on the will of the individual to complete the action in a specific way or in a specific amount of time. Compounding the difficulties is the fact that fatigue can present itself in a fluctuating manner; consequently, an action that is possible at one moment of the day is no longer possible at another, or even the following day. These unforeseeable fluctuations make it difficult to plan one's activities, particularly when they involve other people, again becoming a source of tension and misunderstandings.

Fatigue does not only present itself in its physical component, but can also be cognitive. In this case, the person perceives tiredness on a mental level; on a neuropsychological level, this contributes to decreasing levels of attention, memory, and analytical concentration (problem solving). The descriptions of this symptomatology range from the sensation of having a muffled head, inside a bubble or inside an aquarium, to the reality of being confused, of not being clear on what to do and how to mentally carry out some operations, of not being able to decide between completely banal alternatives.

In this condition, stimuli such as background noise can contribute to one's distraction prompting even greater cerebral exhaustion. An example could be clerical work which involves the use of computers, perhaps in a large "open space" office or in an environment where voices in the background, ringing telephones, comings and goings of people from various offices, are constant factors for one to grapple with. Under these mental conditions, one is consequently less productive or may make mistakes. This last aspect has particularly negative consequences, because it easily leads to developing mistrust in oneself and one's abilities. Anxiety increases, and the doubt of having carried out certain steps correctly or of having done everything that needed to be done to complete a certain task becomes a constant state of being. Meaning one feels forced to review their own operations or asks others to check if everything has been done correctly. While on the one hand, these controls contribute to providing security, on the other they create a sort of dependence on others and the feeling of a lack of autonomy, compounded by self-critical judgments of inadequacy, flaw, and sometimes even uselessness.

Cognitive disorders

Sometimes, fatigue accentuates cognitive disorders, but it is not certain that fatigue and cognitive difficulty always appear together, they may also occur one in the absence of the other. In recent years, the literature has given ample space to the neuropsychological aspects of illness, highlighting how an early evaluation of cognitive disorders is fundamental in order to intervene on cognitive decline (Borghi et al., 2016; Kalb et al., 2018).

Cognitive impairment is a common sign and symptom, yet sometimes overlooked, regardless of the profound effect it has on daily life. The prevalence[3] of cognitive impairment in MS varies through the course of one's lifespan; it can present itself in the early stages of the disease and at a young age, while in older age it may be difficult to distinguish it from other causes (Benedict et al., 2020).

Among the neuropsychological deficits, the one most cited by people and which creates the most emotional distress is memory impairment; it may be verbal or visuospatial memory that is affected. It follows that the subject perceives an absence of control over his own mnemonic abilities, and therefore judges himself to be less efficient than others. The most common problem is the initial difficulty in learning new information. At the beginning of new learning, the person with MS tends to have a need to listen, or repeat the same information several times in order to store it; when this information is acquired, it is recalled to memory in the correct way. This means that from a qualitative point of view the information is stored correctly, but that it takes longer to do this, than in persons who do not have MS. Retrieving information can also be more difficult: one may forget an appointment, where an object was placed, or what another person said during a conversation.

Another cognitive function that is affected is the speed of information processing. In this case there is a slower performance but, if the person is given the time one needs to encode the information, the performance is comparable to that of someone who does not have the disease.

Neuropsychological disorders can be amplified by the presence of fatigue, emotional stress, or a depressed mood. Often their presence undermines self-esteem and the sense of self-efficacy, exacerbating the sense of inadequacy and favoring emotions such as shame, anger, sadness, and guilt.

Since it is estimated that these disorders are present in between 43% and 70% of people with MS (Grzegorski & Losy, 2017), it is of vital importance to take this into serious consideration. Often those who are aware of having some memory, attention or concentration problems tend to be anxious about the future: they project themselves forward in time thinking of themselves as incapable of managing these problems and of "being out of control". Also in this case, beyond specific rehabilitation programs at a cognitive level, it is very useful to teach some exercises of listening to one's breathing and awareness of one's body to increase the level of concentration, thus easing the sense of confusion and mental disorientation (Willekens et al., 2018).

Balance disorders

The presence of anomalies in postural control and gait can appear already in the early stages of the disease. Literature data shows that 50–80% of sufferers have balance and gait dysfunctions, and over 50% fall at least once a year (Cameron & Nilsagard, 2018).

If balance is affected, it is difficult to carry out certain movements, such as walking itself; it is no longer possible to ride a bicycle or dance, and even driving can sometimes be dangerous. One often feels drunk, because they have the sensation of drifting and what one looks at is perceived as constantly moving even if it is a fixed stimulus. For example, if you are sitting in front of the computer, you may have the sensation that the words on the screen are moving, or that the lines of an Excel file are overlapping. To address this symptom, one can appeal to concentration to calibrate one's movements in every detail to feel safer and avoid tripping, falling or worsening the symptom by brisk movements. More complex movements must be broken down into simpler movements that can be performed one at a time. If, for example, one has to get up from the chair and turn around, instead of making the two movements simultaneously the subject learns to first get up, and then, calmly, turn around.

This symptom contributes to feeling more insecure, awkward, and sometimes, it is necessary to make changes to one's clothing in order to sustain one's balance at a secure level. In particular, women can find strategies such as putting their handbag over their shoulder or giving up high heels, preferring more relaxed comfortable shoes. These changes, however, are sometimes particularly difficult to accept because they affect the image that the individual has of oneself. Often these aspects are not even made explicit, because women are ashamed and fear being judged as superficial and too attached to their external image.

Another aspect that often emerges is feeling observed by others and perceiving other people's pity toward oneself. A typical interpretation by patients of other people's perceptions is explained with the phrase: "Poor thing, I'm so sorry!". This judgment, triggered from a person witnessing one's difficulty in balance, unleashes experiences of frustration and emotions such as anger and shame. When this last emotion prevails over the others, avoidance behaviors and behaviors similar to those of one suffering from social phobia can develop.

Generally, the imbalance is visible to others, but sometimes, it is a subjective perception of instability and movement of oneself or objects around one. If, on the one hand, this "invisible" way of presenting the symptom does not lead to social anxiety, on the other, frustration mixes with anger due to having to learn to live with a symptom that no one else recognizes. In many cases, in fact, there are no exercises or manipulations that can help completely solve the problem. People try specific physiotherapy exercises, visit ENT (ear, nose and throat) doctors, even try alternative and complementary therapies, but in some cases, nothing is effective. We therefore feel at the mercy of a symptom that we cannot control; to this is added, as an aggravating factor, the fact that from a neurological point of view there are no detectable indications of worsening, and this determines the thought of not being completely believed or understood by doctors.

Walking disorders

Impaired walking is a common consequence of MS that can lead to substantial limitations in daily activities and compromise one's quality of life. Even enduring one's impairment requires increase in effort and constant adaptation to be able to walk in daily life (Motl & Learmonth, 2014).

In addition to being a very common symptom, walking impairment is also extremely feared by patients from the onset of the disease. In fact, often patients visualize being forced to use a wheelchair in their more or less immediate future, and this thought creates anxiety, anguish, and fear for the course of the disease. Although the association "multiple sclerosis-wheelchair" is in reality much less justified today than in the past, in the patients' vision, it still remains a fearful scenario, and sometimes taken for granted, which risks significantly to affect one's quality of life in the here and now. In fact, it can happen that a person experiences the present with great suffering, even though the disease has been recently diagnosed and the symptoms are mild, due to their fantasies of serious progression with respect to the future.

In the event that walking difficulties arise and it is necessary to introduce an aid such as a crutch, a cane or – a decidedly rarer eventuality in the case of newly diagnosed patients – a walker or wheelchair, psychological resistance frequently emerges. Assistive devices are not seen as aids to be able to maintain as much autonomy as possible when moving, but are experienced as symbols of the inexorable progression of the illness, and therefore avoided. Only a minority of people who need support for mobility have a reasonable psychological adaptation to the use of aids from the beginning. In most patients, a constantly evolving adaptation process is triggered which can be interrupted; transitions from one aid to another can be accompanied by different psychological reactions and it is therefore useful to intervene to facilitate a new accommodation. People may also be forced to use assistive devices on a practical level, but this use can still be associated with considerable emotional distress. Therefore, even if from a behavioral point of view a person uses devices, it is not certain that they are able to remain within their emotional window of tolerance (Siegel, 2010).

One study explored perceptions of walking mobility in people with MS by reporting their reactions after watching themselves walk on video. The study finds that people develop a learned self-awareness of how they walk and what their walking looks like. Acceptance of the reduction in walking function is variable and for this reason the authors underline how self-observation on video can become a tool capable of improving the acceptance of the characteristics of one's walking and coping strategies to promote adaptation (Knox et al., 2020).

Bladder disorders

From a psychological point of view, bladder or sphincter disorder is particularly disabling when it appears at the beginning of the disease process. The person experiences helplessness, frustration, and paralyzing shame over the episode in which they realized they could not control their bladder or sphincters; furthermore, one often lives in fear that this could happen again. Since it is an eventuality that occurs without warning, one fears that it could happen at any moment: one can therefore adopt functional strategies, such as going out with an absorbent pad, or a dysfunctional strategy, such as avoiding drinking for hours or completely avoiding leaving one's home. Those who have had episodes of incontinence often need to be helped to emotionally reconstruct what has happened; otherwise, they will hardly be able to unblock themselves and continue to live a quality life. Bladder retention, on the other hand, which involves incomplete emptying of the bladder with urination, can favor the development of repeated infections which can become complicated and even turn into kidney infections. Intermittent catheterization can be a valid help but, even in this case, accepting an invasive aid, to be introduced inside the body, can be very tiring and emotionally painful.

Furthermore, bladder disorders can be accompanied by intestinal disorders and associated with sexual disorders. All these symptoms are linked to a low quality of life even in newly diagnosed patients. Recognition and adequate treatment of these disorders are necessary to prevent the development of more serious dysfunctions and consequently to maintain a good quality of life (Vitkova et al., 2014).

Vision disorders

Optic neuritis is one of the most frequent symptoms of MS and is often the first symptom to appear; it often represents the reason why the person undergoes the medical tests that will lead to the diagnosis of MS. Optic neuritis manifests itself as a decrease in visual acuity in one eye and is often associated with pain; other times the presence of nystagmus (oscillatory, rhythmic and involuntary movements of the eyeballs) and diplopia (double vision) is found. Recovery of vision can be complete or partial and is facilitated by taking cortisone boluses.

As with other symptoms, due to its sudden onset, it is possible to develop a sense of helplessness and loss of control, sensations that tend to persist if the symptom does not disappear completely. In this case, the symptom takes on the connotation of invisibility, a characteristic discussed previously, but it is very disturbing for the subject, who constantly sees in a blurry or double way, because the eye continually searches for a visual accommodation that does not occur. Driving, looking at a computer screen, or simply looking at an object or person are consequently activities that are both physically and emotionally tiring.

Furthermore, optic neuritis together with the most frequent symptoms at onset – such as paresthesia and numbness in one part of the body – becomes the signal of the fracture between a before and an after: life before the diagnosis in which the image of oneself is characterized by health, and the aftermath, in which the subject deals with the illness and all that it entails.

Depression and anxiety

Depression in people with MS is estimated to have a prevalence of 50%. This prevalence is much higher than other chronic neurological diseases and is three times higher than in the general population (Boeschoten et al., 2017; Carletto et al., 2016). Depression has been considered both a direct consequence of neurological damage and a psychological reaction to illness, with interpretations that remain controversial (Sà, 2008). There is a strong correlation between fatigue and depression and also between depression and anxiety, and these interactions have important implications for one's quality of life. The Goldman Consensus Conference on Depression in MS stated that affective disorders are generally underreported by clinicians and therefore often untreated (McIntosh et al., 2023).

It has been found that non-somatic symptoms of depression (for example: little interest or pleasure in doing things; feeling down, hopeless; experiencing feelings of punishment and failure) are associated with higher levels of anxiety symptoms, and that people with a history of depression may be at higher risk of experiencing anxious states over time (Hartoonian et al., 2002). An additional aspect to consider is that anxiety and depression in MS include overlapping somatic symptoms, such as sleep disturbances, fatigue and difficulty concentrating. Likewise, numbness and tingling, as well as a feeling of unsteadiness, could be attributed to anxiety or neurological symptoms of the illness. Non-somatic symptoms are more linked to the anxiety that arises at the onset of the neurological pathology, while somatic symptoms are predominantly linked to the anxiety that occurs later on the path of one's illness (Hartoonian et al., 2002).

In any case, it is clear that taking care of people who experience states of anxiety or affective disorders, such as depression, by recognizing early on who could benefit from psychological support, is a fundamental aspect and an essential best clinical practice in the context of a multidisciplinary team.

Emotions and thoughts (Federica Graziano)

Managing negative emotions

People suffering from a chronic illness such as MS find themselves in a situation that is by definition unpredictable and fluctuating over time, characterized by multiple symptoms and the prospect of progressive worsening. For this reason, it is normal for them to experience a wide range of negative emotions, which include sadness, fear and anger and all the various shades that they can take on, depending on the circumstances and the course of the disease.

The first studies on the psychological aspects of MS focused primarily on depression (Feinstein, 2011; Sà, 2008). In fact, as just said, it represents a widespread problem among patients with MS, which can affect up to 50% of individuals, even if prevalence estimates are variable, in relation to the specificities of the samples and the criteria considered (Boeschoten et al., 2017). However, using the label "depression" indiscriminately is often misleading. First and foremost, because in many cases, depressive symptoms do not satisfy the diagnostic criteria to identify a real depressive disorder, but rather represent contingent and reactive symptoms with respect to the difficulties of an illness, in a context of general psychological balance (Feinstein et al., 2014).

The varied panorama of emotions that refer to sadness (unhappiness, discouragement, despondency, negative mood, pessimism, distrust, desperation) is characteristic of the experiences of people with MS. Sadness is linked to the changes and the experience of loss that the illness brings with it, in particular the loss of some functions and the modification of the self-image. The sense of guilt is also an experience present in some patients, who tend to attribute to themselves the responsibility for the illness, for its relapse, or for a worsening of the symptoms. It is an irrational thought, often also reinforced from the outside by attitudes of blaming the patient, in turn dictated by defense methods toward a situation that is frightening and that one cannot explain. The sense of guilt is accompanied by a focus on the past, a sense of helplessness and a passive attitude that hinders adaptation to the illness. When a heavily negative mood or a persistent sense of guilt become habitual ways of experiencing an ill condition, risky situations arise for the individual which must be appropriately taken care of. On the contrary, experiences of sadness, if temporary and not very marked, can be considered necessary moments of retreat, functional for distancing oneself from difficulties and useful for developing more adaptive ways to deal with them. Depressive experiences can be signs that appear at particular times, for example, during a relapse or worsening of symptoms, which do not necessarily need to be eliminated immediately. The challenge consists in listening to what one has to say, then translating it into an opportunity for personal growth (Bonino, 2021).

A second psychological problem widespread among people with MS refers to anxiety disorders, which affect a variable percentage, from 15% to 50%, also in this case depending on the samples and the specific criteria used in the individual studies (Boeschoten et al., 2017). The literature also highlights a co-occurrence between anxiety disorders and depressive symptoms (Butler et al., 2016). As already mentioned for depression, even if there is often no diagnosis of anxiety disorder, emotions that refer to one's sense of apprehension and fear are widely spread among people with MS. Fear represents an intense emotion that is activated when faced with a real danger and prepares the individual for a behavioral reaction suited to facing it. It can therefore be considered an important signal that sets defense mechanisms in motion. Anxiety represents a reaction that can be activated in the face of a perceived threat, often in an anticipatory way, persisting over time with different degrees of intensity. The line between fear and anxiety can be blurred, and increasingly, intense levels of anxiety can come to be an actual psychological disorder.

Anxiety is an experience that often characterizes the moment of diagnosis, especially for women (Giordano et al., 2011; Janssen et al., 2003), which can return with every fluctuation of the illness or manifest itself as anticipatory anxiety of future impediments. It is mainly linked to the unpredictability of the disease, to the perception of not having control of the symptoms, to fear of relapses, worsening and disability and the uncertainty of the future. In this regard, some authors talk about specific forms of fear that characterize patients, such as the "fear of relapse" (Khatibi et al., 2020) and the "fear of worsening" (fear of progression; Herschbach et al., 2005).

These are reactive emotional responses, of which people are fully aware, that can negatively impact mood, favoring depressive experiences and a worsening of quality of life (Herschbach et al., 2005; Khatibi et al., 2020). Patients also experience uncertainty and fears in relation to therapies. For example, anxiety linked to the self-administration of some therapies through injection, however used less today (self-injection anxiety; Turner et al., 2009). A patient may fear the often very serious side effects of some therapies or may experience anxiety every time a change is made in the treatment plan and a new, unfamiliar therapy must be introduced. A number of people also report experiences of anxiety every time they have to undergo diagnostic tests, for example, MRI, both due to the type of exam itself and the fear of discovering new lesions. In addition, to the aspects more directly linked to symptoms and treatments, anxiety is also due to the impact the illness has on daily life, work, relationships with family and friends (Butler et al., 2016). In particular, concerns are linked to no longer being able to work as before, being discriminated against at work if the diagnosis is communicated, or losing their job itself. In regard to relationships with others, there is a fear of having to depend on someone and of how others may react to the communication of the diagnosis. Anxiety is also accompanied by other negative emotions, such as embarrassment or shame associated with fear of social stigma (Butler et al., 2016). It is clear that all these aspects can have negative repercussions on the quality of life and must certainly be taken into account when they reach levels of intense suffering for the individual. On the other hand, the emotion of fear and experiences of anxiety must be considered as useful signals to activate response methods that are not based on denial or avoidance, defense mechanisms that are not useful in the long term to cope in adaptive ways to impending difficulties. The greatest challenge for the person with MS is enduring the inevitable state of uncertainty, with the awareness that some aspects of the illness are not controllable, and that therefore it is necessary to deal with inescapable limits. However, within these limits and constraints, possibilities for action are open, setting realistic objectives and developing adequate and effective action strategies (Bonino, 2021).

Among the negative emotions, anger has generally been less investigated in the literature, despite the important unfavorable repercussions that it can have, both on individual well-being and on social relationships. Anger manifests itself mainly as a consequence of an experience of frustration and irritation, linked to the symptoms – in particular fatigue and pain – and to the limitations imposed by the illness, which often make it impossible to engage in the same activities that were carried out before the diagnosis, or they don't allow you to do it at the same pace. This frustration often translates into anger, which the individual directs toward himself or others. In particular, many patients report feeling irritated toward family members, friends or colleagues who often do not understand their difficulties – especially when linked to invisible symptoms that are difficult for an external observer to detect – or, on the contrary, are excessive in their interest and give help, even when not requested. Frustration can also manifest itself toward healthcare personnel, who sometimes do not provide satisfactory answers to the patient or demonstrate poor empathic understanding (Laing et al., 2019).

Anger is a common reaction in the early stages of the disease after communication of the diagnosis (Giordano et al., 2011), although experiences of frustration can recur with each relapse or worsening of the symptoms, situations that put the patient faced with the limitations caused by the illness. If, on the one hand, anger can be considered a normal reaction when it is transitory, on the other, if it transforms into aggression against oneself and others and becomes a habitual modality, it risks having counterproductive effects. Some studies, in particular, have highlighted that anger is linked to a lower quality of life and greater depressive symptoms, while rumination, i.e., a "circular" form of repetitive, passive thinking focused on internal emotional states and their negative consequences (Harrington & Blankenship, 2002), is in turn linked to anxious symptoms. Emotional venting is also not useful in the long term, but risks further aggravating the emotional experience (Laing et al., 2015). For this reason, anger must be recognized, translated into an active perspective and channeled toward realistic objectives that are intended to be pursued effectively. In this way, anger can be overcome and transformed into a strong and energetic drive capable of promoting well-being and adaptation to the illness (Bonino, 2021). Anger transformed in this way can therefore perform a positive function: it can help us understand the limits of a situation, it can transform into a sense of determination and self-confidence and give the right motivation to find alternative ways of achieving one's goals (Harmon-Jones et al., 2010; Litvak et al., 2010).

From emotions to thoughts and from thoughts to emotions

Psychological studies on emotions have long underlined the importance of cognitive evaluation in modulating the physiological response. In particular, emotions are closely associated with physical reactions or physiological states, thoughts and behaviors, and all these aspects influence each other in a circular model of relationship, which represents one of the principles underlying cognitive behavioral therapy (CBT; Beck, 2011). In particular, negative emotions affect bodily reactions, for example, by increasing the sensation of fatigue or pain, and are usually associated with negative thoughts and poorly functional behaviors. Depending on the type of interpretation that the person gives to the association between bodily reaction, emotion, thought and behavior, negative circularities can be established which will tend to feed on themselves. An example of negative circularity can be observed in the following situation.

A patient with MS suddenly wakes up and feels a sensation of pain in their leg and intense tingling (physical reaction). Immediately, a strong worry is activated in them and they experience a state of anxiety (emotion). The patient associates their pain with that experienced in the past during a relapse and thinks they are about to have a new relapse: they will be forced to be hospitalized again and this time they will no longer be able to walk (catastrophic thinking). For several days, they will focus excessively on the body and on the symptoms, they will tend to limit themselves in activities for fear of not being able to complete them (behavior) and this will lead to a further increase in their emotional response.

The same situation can be interpreted and experienced differently, even starting from the same initial bodily reaction, but triggering a positive circularity.

The patient feels a sensation of pain in the leg and intense tingling (physical reaction). This causes them a state of emotional activation, but they think that it is not necessarily the sign of a new relapse: it could be normal symptoms already experienced in the past, with a fluctuating trend (realistic thinking). The fear can be contained, the person feels an emotion of general tranquility and serenity, and carries out daily activities with a remodulation based on the limits posed by the symptom; if the situation persists they will take action to ask the doctor for instructions (adaptive behavior) and as a consequence of this evaluation they experience an overall positive emotional state.

From this example, it is clear how the establishment of a negative circularity can profoundly influence adaptation to the disease, compromising mood and the more general quality of life. The objectives of the cognitive-behavioral approach include making the patient aware of the links that exist between physical reactions, emotions, thoughts, behaviors, and helping one to manage emotions and restructure one's way of thinking, in order to facilitate the establishment of positive circularities.

Restructuring your thoughts and behaviors, in turn, has a positive impact on the emotions and bodily sensations one experiences. Restructuring one's way of thinking means recognizing that sometimes one has dysfunctional thoughts, such as catastrophic thinking ("If I have another relapse, I will end up in a wheelchair"), the tendency to generalize and reach arbitrary conclusions starting from a particular case ("Yesterday I tried to rest to reduce the feeling of fatigue, but it didn't work, so it will never work"), the tendency to consider only the negative sides of a situation and ignore the positive ones ("Today I'm good, but I have symptoms every day, so it won't last") and the tendency to "read other people's minds" and imagine what others might think ("People will think I'm strange because I use a cane"). All these ways of thinking have the characteristics of being automatic, distorted, accepted as such, not questioned, and therefore difficult to deactivate and modify. A change may be possible when one becomes aware of these modalities and try to replace them with more adaptive ones. This in turn will have positive repercussions on emotional experiences and behaviors. The examples of dysfunctional thoughts above could be modified as follows:

> I can't know if I'll have another relapse and I can't live waiting for something to happen when I don't know if it will happen. I will face the demands when they arise.
>
> Yesterday, I tried to rest to reduce the feeling of fatigue, but it didn't work, so I have to plan activities and moments of rest better or try relaxation techniques.
>
> Today I feel good, this makes me feel calm, so I plan activities based on what I feel like doing today.
>
> If I use the cane I may feel a little embarrassed in front of other people, but most of them probably won't even notice and won't think I'm strange.

A further important aspect regarding thought and emotions refers to optimism. On the one hand, it may seem dissonant to talk about optimism in a situation of chronic illness, characterized, as we have seen, by various negative emotions, the experience of pain, uncertainty and unpredictability about the future. Optimism can be defined as an individual's disposition or tendency to have generally favorable expectations for the future (Carver & Scheier, 1994). Various works in the literature have highlighted that optimism is one of the factors that favor adaptation to chronic illness (Fournier et al., 2002; Hurt et al., 2014). In particular, more optimistic people tend to experience lower levels of depression and better psychological and social adaptation to MS (De Ridder et al., 2000; Hart et al., 2008; Moss-Morris et al., 2010). It is plausible that the most optimistic people are able to find heartening aspects even in a challenging situation such as chronic illness, undoubtedly grasping the challenge posed by this specific situation and translating it into a favorable time for further personal development (Pakenham & Cox, 2009, 2012).

In this work, we will always refer to an optimism that is defined as "realistic" or "creative" (Bonino, 2021). It is understood as the ability to respond to impediments with an active attitude being open to change. This ability involves recognizing the limits of a given situation and, within these limits, flexibly seeking strategies to overcome barriers. In particular, this form of productive thinking is contrasted both with defeatist thinking, of which some examples have been illustrated previously (for example, catastrophic thinking), and with illusory thinking. The latter represents a cognitive distortion that does not take reality and its limits into account. For example, a person with MS may think of doing exactly the same things as before, feeling invincible, as if the disease does not exist or has no influence. Cultivating an illusory thought represents a non-adaptive modality in the long term, because the inevitable disillusionment sooner or later leads to colliding with limits and fuels potentially very negative visions of reality. Adhering to a realistic optimism, however, means recognizing the limits, but also the possibilities granted by the disease and using this space for action in a creative way.

Communication (Federica Graziano)

The theme of communication represents a fundamental aspect for the relationships and well-being of individuals, and its role is central when talking about chronic illness. In the condition of illness, some communication difficulties may in fact emerge for the individual which require to be adequately recognized and addressed in order to improve individual psychological well-being.

A dilemma that affects most people with MS is whether to reveal or hide their condition from other people. Since for many patients the symptoms of the disease are not visible on the outside, it is relatively easy to hide one's condition, at least in the initial stages or in any case if the disease remains stationary over time. The person can decide to reveal their condition to and to whom to hide it from. We often decide "not to say" to avoid forms of stigmatization and discrimination, both in social relationships and, above all, in the workplace. On the one hand, it is certainly a stressful situation for the individual, because it involves hiding a part of oneself, on the other hand, as long as the advantages of "not telling" outweigh the disadvantages, this choice produces a feeling of control and is adaptive (Cook et al., 2016). Hiding your condition becomes more difficult and involves greater psychological costs when symptoms become visible or during relapses. After an analysis of the costs and benefits of this communication, the individual can then decide to reveal their condition to some people. The problem of communicating the diagnosis arises above all in the working context, where "not saying" protects against the risk of discrimination or even loss of job, but "saying" allows you to have specific protections, enjoy permissions, and benefit from adjustments in rhythms and working times (Lorefice et al., 2018). In relationships with family and friends, the choice to "say" or "not say" is motivated by various factors. For example, the individual may decide not to communicate their illness to avoid worries for family members, for fear of being a burden, or to avoid compassionate attitudes. One may decide to communicate it only to their relatives or closest friends, or on the contrary to reveal one's condition without problems to everyone. The choice always depends on a set of individual and contextual factors and should be the result of a cost-benefit analysis, which allows the individual to best preserve their psychological well-being.

In addition to the dilemma of "to say" or "not to say", other difficult situations may arise for patients from a communicative point of view. For example, a person may find themselves in the position of having to ask others for help, but give up doing so for fear of being a burden to other people, or because they feel belittled if they do not demonstrate that they are able to be autonomous. In these cases, it is clear how automatic dysfunctional thoughts are activated, of which the individual should become aware in order to be able to adequately restructure them. In other situations, a person may find themself, on the contrary, in a situation in which others give unsolicited help, or behave in ways that the person concerned does not agree with.

To avoid experiences of anger and frustration, in this case too it is important to stop and reflect on the situation and activate effective ways of communicating one's experiences. Through effective and assertive communication, the individual can ask for the kind of help they need and express their requests, thoughts and feelings. Assertive communication consists of being able to express one's needs, feelings, and thoughts in a direct, honest, and appropriate manner, and to defend one's positions without violating the rights of others (Moss-Morris et al., 2010). The assertive person is able to communicate appropriately depending on the interlocutor, in an open, direct and frank manner. Assertive communication differs from both aggressive and passive communication. While aggressive communication can be defined as the affirmation of oneself "against" the other, assertive communication consists in the affirmation of oneself "in respect" of the other, while in passive communication, the individual simply waits for things to happen, in assertive communication the attitude is active and proactive.

Assertive communication, which is fundamental in all social relationships, is also essential in the relationship with healthcare professionals in the specific case of a person with MS. Many patients report how healthcare staff often do not demonstrate empathetic understanding of their struggles, or do not provide them with clear and understandable answers (Laing et al., 2019). Communicating assertively with healthcare professionals means clearly expressing one's requests, formulating one's doubts, demanding clear and exhaustive answers, in a real collaborative relationship between patient and doctor, which in turn positively affects adherence to therapies, as well as one's psychological well-being (Bonino, 2021). In this regard, studies underline the importance for patients and their families to have clear and comprehensive information on the disease, symptoms and treatments (Box et al., 2003). The possibility of having satisfactory information promotes a sense of control over the disease, the use of more effective coping strategies, and the reduction of anxious and depressive experiences (Lode et al., 2007; Messmer Uccelli et al., 2013).

Finally, the ability to communicate effectively and assertively makes it possible to benefit from a social support network, an aspect that promotes a better quality of life and reduces stress levels, anxiety disorders and depressive experiences (Dennison et al., 2011; Lode et al., 2009). Helping people to communicate effectively in relationships is therefore one of the aspects capable of promoting the process of adaptation to this illness.

Toward acceptance of the disease: A continuous adaptation process (Federica Graziano and Emanuela Calandri)

The expression "acceptance of the illness", often used when talking about chronic illness, must not be understood as synonymous with "resignation" or "renunciation", nor should it make us think of something passive and given once and for all. Instead, it is a question of accepting illness as one's reality and life condition, with its limits but also with its opportunities, in a perspective of personal fulfillment and development (Bonino, 2021). Acceptance is the fruit of a successful adaptation to the conditions of illness and its evolution over time. Consequently, to promote acceptance, it is necessary to work on the process of "continuous adaptation" to the disease in which, as mentioned, the patient has an active role. Adaptation to the multiple difficulties imposed by the disease, both immediately after diagnosis and following, implying a continuous search for a new situation of balance (Moss-Morris, 2013). Adaptation includes the ability to be flexible and open to change and live in the present moment, engaging in what is possible, to try to preserve a reasonable quality of life (Moss-Morris et al., 2010). Adaptation is a continuous process; in a first phase, it is adaptation to the diagnosis, and then, along the course of the disease, there are various adaptations to the relapses and progression of the disease. At some times, a person will successfully cope with the challenge, at other times they will feel that they cannot cope and may actually have difficulties. All this is part of the fluctuating trend of the illness, which requires continuous adaptations. However, only by adaptively addressing the various challenges that this illness poses, the individual can translate this critical experience into an opportunity for growth and development (Hendry & Kloep, 2002).

Adaptation is a goal that can be achieved through all the methods mentioned in the previous paragraphs.

First, redefining one's identity, giving meaning to life with chronic illness and reformulating one's significant goals from time to time, defining effective strategies to achieve them, are central factors that can promote a person's adaptation to MS. While these three constructs have generally been considered separately in the literature, in the theoretical model underlying the intervention presented here they are considered aspects that are closely connected to each other. As already mentioned in the previous chapter, they interact and influence each other in a circular way: in particular, the sense of self-efficacy allows the achievement of significant, coherent and meaningful objectives, in which to realize one's identity (Bonino, 2021).

Second, a central role is played by the ability to manage symptoms and one's relationship with the body. Faced with uncontrollable symptoms, adaptation also consists of accepting what cannot be changed and trying to reduce the impact that one's illness has on everyday life.

Third, emotions and thoughts play a crucial role. As mentioned, MS brings with it a set of negative emotions and these experiences represent continuous challenges. Part of adapting is recognizing these negative emotions, giving them a name and trying to manage them, without being overwhelmed by them. Recognizing the mutual influences between emotions, thoughts, physical sensations and behaviors can pave the way to a self-awareness that can undoubtedly improve one's quality of life and well-being.

Last, but not least, the ability to communicate with others effectively and assertively allows you to express your thoughts and feelings and allows you to count on social support, therefore playing a central role in adaptation to chronic illness.

It is therefore on each of these aspects that the psychological support intervention aimed at newly diagnosed patients described in the following chapter focuses upon.

Notes

1 For an in-depth and up-to-date discussion on the topic of identity in relation to multiple sclerosis, see Graziano et al. (2025). Multiple sclerosis and identity: a mixed-methods systematic review. *Disability and Rehabilitation*, 47:9, 2199–2216. https://doi.org/10. 1080/09638288.2024.2392039
2 Since it is not the aim of this book to give an exhaustive description of the symptoms of multiple sclerosis, in the following paragraphs some of them will be described, with particular attention to those most frequent in people who have recently received the diagnosis.
3 In medical statistics, "prevalence" means the proportion of events present in a specific population at a given moment.

References

Antonovsky, A. (1987). *Unraveling the mystery of health*. Jossey Bass Publishers.

Arnett, J. J. (2000). Emerging adulthood: A theory of development from the late teens through the twenties. *American Psychologist*, *55*, 469–480.

Aujoulat, I. (2007). *L'empowerment des patients atteints de maladie chronique. Des processus multiples: auto-détermination, auto-efficacité, sécurité et cohérence identitaire [The empowerment of chronically ill patients. Multiple processes: self-determination, self-efficacy, confidence and identity coherence]*, PhD Thesis, Université Catholique de Louvain, Ecole de santé publique, Unité d'éducation pour la santé RESO.

Baltes, P. B. (1997). On the incomplete architecture of human ontogenesis: Selection, optimization and compensation as foundations of developmental theory. *American Psychologist*, *52*, 366–381.

Bandura, A. (1997). *Self-efficacy. The exercise of control*. Freeman and Company.

Beck, J. S. (2011). *Cognitive behavior therapy, second edition: Basics and beyond*. The Guilford Press.

Benedict, R. H. B., Amato, M. P., DeLuca, J., & Geurts, J. J. G. (2020). Cognitive impairment in multiple sclerosis: Clinical management, MRI, and therapeutic avenues. *The Lancet Neurology*, *19*, 860–871.

Boeschoten, R. E., Braamse, A. M. J., Beekman, A. T. F., Cuijpers, P., van Oppen, P., Dekker, J., & Uitdehaag, B. M. J. (2017). Prevalence of depression and anxiety in multiple sclerosis: A systematic review and meta-analysis. *Journal of the Neurological Sciences*, *372*, 331–341.

Bonino, S. (2021). *Coping with chronic illness. Theories, issues and lived experiences.* Routledge.

Borghi, M., Carletto, S., Ostacoli, L., Scavelli, F., Pia, L., Pagani, M., Bertolotto, A., Malucchi, S., Signori, A., & Cavallo, M. (2016). Decline of neuropsychological abilities in a large sample of patients with multiple sclerosis: A two-year longitudinal study. *Frontiers in Human Neuroscience, 10*, Article 282.

Bosma, H. A., & Kunnen, E. S. (2001). Determinants and mechanisms in ego identity development: A review and synthesis. *Developmental Review, 21*, 39–66.

Bottaccioli, F., & Bottaccioli, A. G. (2020). *Psycho neuro endocrine immunology and science of the integrated care. The manual.* Edra.

Box, V., Hepworth, M., & Harrison, J. (2003). Identifying information needs of people with multiple sclerosis. *Nursing Times, 99*, 32–36.

Breakwell, G. (1983). *Threatened identities.* Wiley.

Butler, E., Matcham, F., & Chalder, T. (2016). A systematic review of anxiety amongst people with multiple sclerosis. *Multiple Sclerosis and Related Disorders, 11*, 145–168.

Cameron, C., & Nilsagard, Y. (2018). Balance, gait, and falls in multiple sclerosis. *Handbook of Clinical Neurology, 159*, 237–250.

Carletto, S., Borghi, M., Francone, D., Scavelli, F., Bertino, G., Cavallo, M., Malucchi, S., Bertolotto, A., Oliva, F., & Ostacoli, L. (2016). The efficacy of a mindfulness based intervention for depressive symptoms in patients with multiple sclerosis and their caregivers: Study protocol for a randomized controlled clinical trial. *BMC Neurology, 6*, Article 7.

Carver, C. S., & Scheier, M. F. (1994). Optimism and health-related cognition: What variables actually matter? *Psychology and Health, 9*, 191–195.

Charmaz, K. (1983). Loss of self: A fundamental form of suffering in the chronically ill. *Sociology of Health and Illness, 5*, 168–195.

Cook, J. E., Germano, A. L., & Stadler, G. (2016). An exploratory investigation of social stigma and concealment in patients with multiple sclerosis. *International Journal of Multiple Sclerosis Care, 18*, 78–84.

De Ceuninck van Capelle, A., Visser, L. H., & Vosman, F. (2016). Multiple sclerosis (MS) in the life cycle of the family: An interpretative phenomenological analysis of the perspective of persons with recently diagnosed MS. *Families, Systems and Health, 34(*4), 435–440.

Dennison, L., Moss-Morris, R., & Chalder, T. (2009). A review of psychological correlates of adjustment in patients with multiple sclerosis. *Clinical Psychology Review, 29*, 141–153.

Dennison, L., Yardley, L., Devereux, A., & Moss-Morris, R. (2011). Experiences of adjusting to early stage multiple sclerosis. *Journal of Health Psychology, 16*, 478–488.

De Ridder, D., Schreurs, K., & Bensing, J. (2000). The relative benefits of being optimistic: Optimism as a coping resource in multiple sclerosis and Parkinson's disease. *British Journal of Health Psychology, 5*, 141–155.

Di Cara, M., Lo Buono, V., Corallo, F., Cannistraci, C., Rifici, C., Sessa, E., D'Aleo, G., Bramanti, P., & Marino, S. (2019). Body image in multiple sclerosis patients: A descriptive review. *Neurological Sciences, 40*, 923–928.

Edwards, R. G., Barlow, J., & Turner, A. P. (2008). Experiences of diagnosis and treatment among people with multiple sclerosis. *Journal of Evaluation in Clinical Practice, 14*, 460–464.

Eriksson, M., & Lindstrom, B. (2006). Antonovsky's sense of coherence scale and the relation with health: A systematic review. *Journal of Epidemiology and Community Health, 60*, 376–381.

Feinstein, A. (2011). Multiple sclerosis and depression. *Multiple Sclerosis, 17*, 1276–1281.

Feinstein, A., Magalhaes, S., Richard, J. F., Audet, B., & Moore, C. (2014). The link between multiple sclerosis and depression. *Nature Reviews Neurology, 10(*9), 507–517.

Ferrier, S., Dunlop, N., & Blanchard, C. (2010). The role of outcome expectations and self-efficacy in explaining physical activity behaviors of individuals with multiple sclerosis. *Behavioral Medicine, 36*, 7–11.

Finlay, L. (2003). The intertwining of body, self and world: A phenomenological study of living with recently-diagnosed multiple sclerosis. *Journal of Phenomenological Psychology, 34*, 157–178.

Ford, D. H., & Lerner, R. M. (1992). *Developmental systems theory: An integrative approach.* Sage Publications, Inc.

Fournier, M., de Ridder, D., & Bensing, J. (2002). Optimism and adaptation to chronic disease: The role of optimism in relation to self-care options of type 1 diabetes mellitus, rheumatoid arthritis and multiple sclerosis. *British Journal of Health Psychology, 7*, 409–432.

Frankl, V. E. (1946). *Man's search for meaning. An introduction to logotherapy.* Beacon Press.

Frankl, V. E. (2011). *The unheard cry for meaning. Psychotherapy and humanism.* Simon & Schuster.

Fraser, C., Hadjimichael, O., & Vollmer, T. (2001). Predictors of adherence to copaxone therapy in individuals with relapsing remitting multiple sclerosis. *Journal of Neuroscience Nursing, 33*, 231–239.

Giordano, A., Granella, F., Lugaresi, A., Martinelli, V., Trojano, M., Confalonieri, P., Radice, D., & Solari, A. (2011). Anxiety and depression in multiple sclerosis patients around diagnosis. *Journal of Neurological Sciences, 307*, 86–91.

Grzegorski, T., & Losy, J. (2017). Cognitive impairment in multiple sclerosis - A review of current knowledge and recent research. *Reviews in Neuroscience, 28*, 845–860.

Gullvi, F., Ek, A. C., & Söderhamn, O. (2003). Lived experience of MS-related fatigue- a phenomenological interview study. *International Journal of Nursing Studies, 40*, 707–717.

Harmon-Jones, E., Peterson, C. K., & Harmon-Jones, C. (2010). Anger, motivation, and asymmetrical frontal cortical activations. In M. Potegal (Ed.), *International handbook of anger* (pp. 61–78). Springer.

Harrington, J. A., & Blankenship, V. (2002). Ruminative thoughts and their relation to depression and anxiety. *Journal of Applied Social Psychology, 32*(3), 465–485.

Hart, S. L., Vella, L., & Mohr, D. C. (2008). Relationships among depressive symptoms, benefit-finding, optimism, and positive affect in multiple sclerosis patients after psychotherapy for depression. *Health Psychology, 27*, 230–238.

Hartoonian, N., Terrill, A. L., Hendry, L. B., & Kloep, M. (2002). *Lifespan development. Resources, challenges and risks.* Thomson Learning.

Hendry, L. B., & Kloep, M. (2002). *Lifespan development. Resources, challenges and risks.* Thomson Learning, trad.it.

Herschbach, P., Berg, P., Dankert, A., Duran, G., Engst-Hastreiter, U., Waadt, S., Ukat, R., & Henrich, G. (2005). Fear of progression in chronic diseases: Psychometric properties of the fear of progression questionnaire. *Journal of Psychosomatic Research, 58*, 505–511.

Holman, H., & Lorig, K. (2004). Patient self-management: A key to effectiveness and efficiency in care of chronic disease. *Public Health Reports, 119*, 239–243.

Hurt, C. S., Burn, D. J., Hindle, J., Samuel, M., Wilson, K., & Brown, R. G. (2014). Thinking positively about chronic illness: An exploration of optimism, illness perceptions And well-being in patients with Parkinson's disease. *British Journal of Health Psychology, 19*, 363–379.

Irvine, H., Davidson, C., Hoy, K., & Lowe-Strong, A. (2009). Psychosocial adjustment to multiple sclerosis: Exploration of identity redefinition. *Disability and Rehabilitation, 31*, 599–606.

Janssen, A. C. J. W., van Doorn, P. A., de Boer, J. B., van der Meche', F. G. A., Passchier, J., & Hintzen, R. Q. (2003). Impact of recently diagnosed multiple sclerosis on quality of life, anxiety, depression, and distress of patients and partners. *Acta Neurologica Scandinavica, 108*, 389–395.

Kalb, R., Beier, M., Benedict Ralph, H. B., Charvet, L., Costello, K., Feinstein, A., Gingold, G., Goverover, Y., Halper, J., Harris, C., Lori Kostich, L., Krupp, L., Lathi, E., LaRocca, N., Thrower, B., & DeLuca, J. (2018). Recommendations for cognitive screening and management in multiple sclerosis care. *Multiple Sclerosis, 13*, 1665–1680.

Khatibi, A., Moradi, N., Rahbari, N., Salehi, T., & Dehghani, M. (2020). Development and validation of fear of relapse scale for relapsing-remitting multiple sclerosis: Understanding stressors in patients. *Frontiers in Psychiatry, 11*, Article 226.

Knox, K. B., Clay, L., Stuart-Kobitz, K., & Nickel, D. (2020). Perspectives on walking from people with multiple sclerosis and reactions to video self-observation. *Disability and Rehabilitation, 42*, 211–218.

Laing, C. M., Cooper, C. L., Summers, F., Lawrie, L., O'Flaherty, S., & Phillips, L. H. (2019). The nature of anger in people with multiple sclerosis: A qualitative study. *Psychology & Health, 35*, 824–837.

Laing, C. M., Phillips, L. H., Cooper, C. L., Hosie, J. A., & Summers, F. (2015). Anger, quality of life and mood in multiple sclerosis. *Journal of Multiple Sclerosis, 2*, 127–132.

Litvak, P. M., Lerner, J. S., Tiedens, L. Z., & Shonk, K. (2010). Fuel in the fire: How anger impacts judgment and decision-making. In M. Potegal (Ed.), *International handbook of anger* (pp. 287–310). Springer.

Lode, K., Bru, E., Klevan, G., Myhr, K. M., Nyland, H., & Larsen, J. P. (2009). Depressive symptoms and coping in newly diagnosed patients with multiple sclerosis. *Multiple Sclerosis, 15*, 638–643.

Lode, K., Larsen, J. P., Bru, E., Klevan, G., Myhr, K. M., & Nyland, H. (2007). Patient information and coping styles in multiple sclerosis. *Multiple Sclerosis, 13*, 792–799.

Lorefice, L., Fenu, G., Frau, J., Coghe, G., Marrosu, M. G., & Cocco, E. (2018). The impact of visible and invisible symptoms on employment status, work and social functioning in multiple sclerosis. *Work, 60*, 263–270.

Magnusson, D., & Stattin, H. (2006). *The person in context: A holistic interactionistic approach*. In W. Damon, & R. M. Lerner (Eds.), *Handbook of child psychology*, VI ed, Vol. 1, pp. 400–464). Wiley.

McIntosh, G. E., Liu, E. S., Allan, M., & Grech, L. B. (2023). Clinical practice guidelines for the detection and treatment of depression in multiple sclerosis: A systematic review. *Neurology: Clinical Practice, 13*(3), e200154.

Messmer Uccelli, M., Traversa, S., Trojano, M., Viterbo, R. G., Ghezzi, A., & Signori, A. (2013). Lack of information about multiple sclerosis in children can impact parents' sense of competency and satisfaction within the couple. *Journal of the Neurological Sciences, 15*, 100–105.

Miller, P., & Soundy, A. (2017). The pharmacological and non-pharmacological interventions for the management of fatigue related multiple sclerosis. *Journal of Neurological Sciences, 381*, 41–54.

Moss-Morris, R. (2013). Adjusting to chronic illness: Time for a unified theory. *British Journal of Health Psychology, 18*, 681–686.

Moss-Morris, R., Dennison, L., & Chalder, T. (2010). *Supportive Adjustment for Multiple Sclerosis (saMS). An eight-week CBT programme manual*. Multiple Sclerosis Society, University of Southampton and King's College London. https://www.bl.uk/collection-items/supportive-adjustment-for-multiple-sclerosis-sams-an-eightweek-cbt-programme-manual#

Motl, R. W., & Learmonth, Y. C. (2014). Neurological disability and its association with walking impairment in multiple sclerosis: Brief review. *Neurodegenerative Disease Management, 4*, 491–500.

Pakenham, K. I. (2007). Making sense of multiple sclerosis. *Rehabilitation Psychology, 52*, 380–389.

Pakenham, K. I., & Cox, S. (2009). The dimensional structure of benefit finding in multiple sclerosis and relations with positive and negative adjustment: A longitudinal study. *Psychology and Health, 24*, 373–393.

Pakenham, K. I., & Cox, S. (2012). The nature of caregiving in children of a parent with multiple sclerosis from multiple sources and the associations between caregiving activities and youth adjustment overtime. *Psychology and Health, 27*, 324–346.

Paterson, B. L. (2001). The shifting perspectives model of chronic illness. *Journal of Nursing Scholarship, 33*, 21–26.

Porges, S. W. (2011). *The polyvagal theory: Neurophysiological foundations of emotions, attachment, communication, self-regulation.* W.W. Norton & Company.

Sà, M. J. (2008). Psychological aspects of multiple sclerosis. *Clinical Neurology and Neurosurgery, 110*, 868–877.

Schmitt, M. M., Goverover, Y., Deluca, J., & Chiaravalloti, N. (2014). Self-efficacy as a predictor of self-reported physical, cognitive, and social functioning in multiple sclerosis. *Rehabilitation Psychology, 59*, 27–34.

Sharon, T. (2015). Constructing adulthood: Markers of adulthood and well-being among emerging adults. *Emerging Adulthood, 4*, 161–167.

Siegel, D. (2010). *The mindful therapist. A Clinician's guide to mindsight and neural integration.* W.W. Norton & Co. Inc.

Solaro, C., Trabucco, E., & Messmer Uccelli, M. (2013). Pain and multiple sclerosis: Pathophysiology and treatment. *Current Neurology and Neuroscience Report, 13*, Article 320.

Stevens, S. D., Thompson, N. R., & Sullivan, A. B. (2019). Prevalence and correlates of body image dissatisfaction in patients with multiple sclerosis. *International Journal of Multiple Sclerosis Care, 21*, 207–213.

Tabuteau-Harrison, S. L., Haslam, C., & Mewse, A. J. (2016). Adjusting to living with multiple sclerosis: The role of social groups. *Neuropsychological Rehabilitation, 26*, 36–59.

Tihanyi, B. T., Ferentzi, E., Beissner, F., & Köteles, F. (2018). The neuropsychophysiology of tingling. *Counsciusness and Cognition, 58*, 97–110.

Toombs, S. K. (1992). *The body in multiple sclerosis: A patient's perspective.* In D. Leder (Ed.), *The body in medical thought and practice* (pp. 127–137). Springer Link.

Turner, A. P., Williams, R. M., Sloan, A. P., & Haselkorn, J. K. (2009). Injection anxiety remains a long-term barrier to medication adherence in multiple sclerosis. *Rehabilitation Psychology, 54*, 116–121.

van der Meide, H., Teunissen, T., Collard, P., Visse, M., & Visser, L. H. (2018). The mindful body: A phenomenology of the body with multiple sclerosis. *Qualitative Health Research, 28*, 2239–2249.

Vitkova, M., Rosenberger, J., Krokavcova, M., Szilasiova, J., Gdovinova, Z., Groothoff, J. W., & van Dijk, J. P. (2014). Health related quality of life in multiple sclerosis patients with bladder, bowel and sexual dysfunction. *Disability and Rehabilitation, 36*, 987–92.

Weinreich, P., & Saunderson, W. (2003). *Analysing identity: Cross-cultural, societal and clinical contexts.* Routledge.

Willekens, B., Perrotta, G., Cras, P., & Cools, N. (2018). Into the moment: Does mindfulness affect biological pathways in multiple sclerosis? *Frontiers in Behavioral Neuroscience, 12*, Article 103.

Wilski, M., & Tasiemski, T. (2016). Illness perception, treatment beliefs, self-esteem, and self-efficacy as correlates of self-management in multiple sclerosis. *Acta Neurologica Scandinavica, 133*, 338–345.

3 The intervention meeting by meeting

Martina Borghi

General guidelines

Before we begin: Enrollment

The recruitment of potential participants who have been recently diagnosed with multiple sclerosis (MS) (no more than three years) to access the path dedicated to newly diagnosed individuals, was done by engaging three complementary methods.

The first consists in the direct reporting of newly diagnosed patients, by doctors and nurses, to the person in charge of collecting the names.

The second method involves a meticulous check, again by the person in charge, of the records of all patients discharged from the neurology department and of the diary with appointments for the new starts of therapy, in order to be sure that all the names have been collected.

The third method consists of self-reporting by people through an information leaflet in which the initiative is advertised and which can be found on the notice-board at the CReSM clinics.

At this time, each newly diagnosed person is contacted personally (mostly via telephone) to briefly explain what the group process consists of and to request their email address to send the invitation to join the group's journey. Then after, each potential participant receives a personal letter of invitation via email, signed by the director of the CReSM and the scientific manager of the project, and a map to reach the meeting place.

In our specific case, these multiple channels of sending possibilities serve to ensure that truly all people who receive the diagnosis of MS are approached. In fact, given the high number of patients that CReSM collects as a regional reference center for Piedmont, it is necessary to diversify the possibilities of access to this dedicated path. Each working reality can have different needs; it may therefore be sufficient for the center staff to send a referral, or for the psychologist leading the group to identify another effective strategy for recruitment, different from those listed above.

Preparation for meetings

The people who participate in the meetings are divided into groups based on age. The optimal subdivisions are 20–35 years, 36–45 years and 46–65 years. In this way,

DOI: 10.4324/9781003484400-3

groups are made up of people who share similar development tasks. This subdivision also promotes the sense of belonging to the group, the understanding of each other's experiences, and the sharing of experiences related to the illness. Regarding the number of participants, experience shows that the optimal number is eight people.

Upon arrival, participants are welcomed into the room dedicated to meetings, inside which the chairs are arranged in a circle to facilitate the interaction and there is a flip chart used by the psychologist to write the guiding questions and note everyone's answers. The care dedicated to the space in which the psychological intervention takes place pursues the objective of building a climate that facilitates communication and the sharing of problems, stimulating cohesion between members in an environment not characterized from a health point of view. A place therefore which does not directly refer to the illness but which welcomes and gives space to the care of the person through the contents of the meetings, the relationships created between the participants within a pleasant and hospitable environment. Even the break in the middle of the meeting, in which drinks are shared, not only responds to the need for a moment of rest but helps maintain a relaxed and comfortable atmosphere.

The first meeting lasts two and a half hours; all the following two hours.

All group meetings are conducted by the team psychologist who have been entrusted with this undertaking. The scientific manager of the intervention project participates only in the first meeting, limited to the time necessary for the presentation of the initiative. An observer is also present in all meetings, a silent presence who does not intervene. In the second part of the seventh meeting, a neurologist responsible for CReSM also participates.

An overview of group meetings

The group is offered a psychological intervention aimed first of all at improving the reorganization of one's identity, at giving a new meaning to the experience of life with illness, at increasing the feeling of self-efficacy and, subsequently, at improving the ability to manage both symptoms, emotional states and stress, and communication with others.

Each meeting has a central theme to be explored and analyzed in these specific areas: emotional relationships, family and friends, work and free time.

Each meeting begins with a short breathing exercise, a body relaxation technique useful for stabilizing presence in the here and now, which can also be used independently at home, given to the written instructions provided.

In the first meeting, we work on the changes one's identity has undergone and perhaps undergoing as well, due to the alterations introduced by MS in a person's life. Specifically, guided reflection leads participants to think about how they lived their emotional relationships, social life, work and free time before the diagnosis and what the changes are in these areas after the diagnosis.

In the second meeting, the restructuring of identity is explored in depth by focusing attention on what gave meaning to life before the diagnosis – that is, what was important, what made one feel fulfilled, what one fought for – and on what in the present can give it meaning and make it feel worth living, considering the changes that MS has introduced in its different areas.

In the third meeting, we work on the feeling of self-efficacy, defined as the sense of security that the person experiences when one knows how to deal with a situation and how to achieve what one has set out to do: thanks to it, the individual knows one's own resources and those of the context, one knows where to find them and how to exploit them, one knows which strategies to use. The steps to be taken to achieve one's specific objectives are consequently examined, with particular attention to the subsequent evaluation of the results and any further adjustments to be made.

After examining how to set achievable goals and how to achieve them, the fourth meeting is where the relationships between emotions, thoughts, physical sensations and actions are analyzed. The aim is to increase the ability to manage negative emotions and moods, promote positive ones and avoid the establishment of vicious cycles between negative thoughts on the one hand and destructive emotions and physical sensations on the other.

The fifth meeting is dedicated to the theme of communication with others, both in significant personal relationships from an emotional or work point of view (family, friends, colleagues, employer), and with those in healthcare personnel, particularly with the neurologist, who deals with the disease. Emphasis is placed on communication as a tool for verbalizing one's needs and experiences and therefore on the importance of implementing effective and clear communication in which manipulations and distortions are limited as much as possible.

The follow-up meeting (sixth meeting) is held six months after the fifth; it has the aim of retracing together the path taken to evaluate any changes made and verify which aspects settled most easily and which ones the participants require to be strengthened.

Finally, one year after the fifth meeting, an in-depth meeting is held (focus group, seventh meeting) with the aim of receiving feedback on the experience gained and identifying the strengths and weaknesses of the project. This allows for an evaluation of whether to keep the structure identical or modify it to improve the organization of the meetings and the topics covered, with adjustments aimed at improving the quality of the proposed intervention path. Part of the time is dedicated to dialogue with the neurologist responsible for CReSM.

Let us now look in depth at the psychological intervention process, meeting by meeting.

First meeting

The foundation of the group, the moment of diagnosis and the start of reflection on one's identity

As in every group journey that begins, the first meeting is always full of expectations and implicit questions from the participants. If on the one hand the meeting of several people arouses curiosity and reassurance, due to the sense of commonality with those who share the same experience, on the other hand some are afraid of not

---

Box 3.1   Meeting 1 – the foundation of the group, the moment of diagnosis and the reflection upon one's identity

Introduction (1.)

- Welcome and presentation by the psychologist facilitator
- Presentation of the project by the scientific manager
- Completing the *Me and my life* questionnaire
- Delivery of the handout
- Presentation of the observer and explanation of their role
- Sharing some rules (confidentiality, punctuality, how to notify if late or absent, pause in the middle of the meeting, willingness to address one another, etc.)
- Presentation of the participants (without request narratives related to MS): what is your name, where and with whom do you live, what you do in life and what you like to do

Contents and topics (2.)

- Fractional breathing
- "What emotions did I feel at the time of diagnosis?" (use of images to describe emotions)
- "What emotions do I feel now?" (use of images to describe emotions)
- Write the answer to the question "Who am I?" in the appropriate handout for yourself

Conclusion (3.)

- Summary of contents emerged from the part of the psychologist
- Invitation to carry out the "homework", see in Appendix 1
- Fractional breathing

---

being able to feel at ease within the group. Specifically, there is a frequent fear of meeting people with a disability greater than one's own, therefore having to deal with the evolution of the illness or with some problem or symptom of which one is not aware. This aspect is inevitable and is indeed a fundamental part of the process of understanding and recognizing the heterogeneous manifestations and different symptoms of this illness. It is critically important that people can discuss their experiences in this initial period in which everything is new and a cause for fear and confusion. Knowing that someone else has also experienced the same symptoms, or had a similar onset to yours, represents reassurance and means feeling less alone. But even when the other person presents different physical symptoms, the person perceives a sense of commonality and closeness with those they have just met, since they already share significant experiences, such as the first relapse and the emotions associated with it.

The first meeting opens with the presentation of the intervention project and the psychological path by Silvia Bonino, who leaves the group after finishing. The aim is to explain how the initiative was born, on which theoretical–clinical assumptions it is based and what objectives we want to achieve. Furthermore, the advantages that group meetings represent compared to individual sessions are highlighted, and the difficulties that group sessions can entail are also anticipated, always with the intention of normalizing any negative sensations that participants may experience. It is also explained that the intervention is subject to continuous research activity, in order to better understand its effectiveness, and that this will take the form of proposing questionnaires to participants, the compilation of which requires everyone's collaboration. Silvia Bonino's introduction is an extremely precious added value as the participants listen to a professional in the psychological area who initiates group work by combining theoretical knowledge and personal experience (see point 1 of Box 3.2 *Points and tips for the facilitator*, in which useful insights are reported in numerical order).

After this introduction, the facilitator delivers the *Me and my life* questionnaire, specifically constructed to investigate the variables that will be the fulcrum of the path and to evaluate the outcomes of the latter.

Subsequently, the facilitator gives some indications to better orient oneself in the space and define some important rules of participation in the group. The information provided relates to the start and end times of meetings, the break that takes place halfway through the meeting, and the location of the bathrooms.

The facilitator continues with a brief explanation of how the sessions will take place: there will always be an exercise of relaxation and listening to breathing, which will mark the "entry" into the group; participants are given a folder containing handout stating the outline of the meetings, the materials used and the "homework" (see Appendix 1). It is explained that to achieve the objectives the active participation of the participants is essential and that the facilitator will use what is said by the individual to underscore, deepening some concepts and convey what is said in psychological terms.

Finally, the facilitator emphasizes the importance of confidentiality with respect to the contents explained by the participants and the need for nothing to be reported to other people, such as family, friends or acquaintances. Confidentiality is imperative to facilitate an atmosphere of sharing and discussion free from judgment, in which everyone can express themselves fully, knowing that the group space is protected and respected.

Afterward, the facilitator begins the presentation of the participants and the constitution of the group in relational terms. The facilitator herself introduces herself first, giving basic and "neutral" information such as her name, where she comes from, how long she has been working in the field of MS. The presentation ends with positive information, which has the value of a personal resource: what you "like" or what you "like to do". What you "like" can be your pet, a favorite food, etc.; what you "like to do" can be an activity such as listening to a certain type of music, cooking, a hobby, a sport, etc. The presentation mode can be modified according to the sensitivity of each facilitator. What is important is to have clear some basic elements that facilitate the work (see point 2 of Box 3.2). The facilitator then leaves the floor and the presentation to the participants.

Now continuing, the facilitator introduces the observer and explains the role the observer will have within the group: a discreet and silent presence whose objective is to transcribe the contents that emerged during the meeting and keep a written record of the dynamics that move within of each group (see Appendix 3, *Observation grid of group meetings*).

Once the presentation round is over, the facilitator introduces the practice of relaxation and breathing, called "fractional breathing" (tracing *How to do relaxation exercises at home* and *How to learn to relax*, see Appendix 1), which is the exercise with which all group meetings will begin. Including this activity at the beginning of the meeting allows participants to learn a simple way to relax that they can self-administer at home; furthermore, it is an important ritual of entry into the group, through which everything that does not concern the group path is left out and through which the space for self-reflection is protected, beginning with from greater bodily awareness.

We then get to the heart of the contents of the first meeting, by introducing the sharing of emotions felt both at the time of diagnosis and currently, discussing each. Participants are then asked to choose an image, among those proposed, which can be representative of their feelings (see point 3 of Box 3.2). These images are a tool chosen to help participants talk about their feelings, referring first to the moment of diagnosis followed by the present.

The images proposed come mainly from newspaper clippings with photographs relating to nature and minimally from advertising images, in order to give the widest possibility of being able to identify themselves (see Appendix 2, *The words of the participants*). Although there are many images, some are chosen more often than others. One of these is the photo of a man on the edge of a precipice, highlighting the emotion of fear and the sensation that a chasm has opened under one's feet. Another is a spider's web, which is associated with a sense of helplessness and the perception of being trapped, with no way out. Then, there are images of thunderstorms, which correspond to the internal disturbance felt at the moment of diagnosis, to the perception of confusion and profound upheaval. Other images are those of the stormy or calm sea, which describe the disorientation and loneliness that can accompany the moment of diagnosis; a foggy landscape instead highlights the worry and anxiety due to the absence of a clear and positive vision of the future. More rarely, images emerge that express anger (such as the image of an animal attacking prey, or the image of a stormy sky). Sometimes, the choice of image emphasizes the sense of closeness to a loved one and a state of affiliation (for example, an animal with its own puppy), indicating a regression to an earlier stage of development. Finally, some images of tidy and delicate landscapes describe the communication of the diagnosis as a moment of greater calm and clarity, because a name is finally given to the symptoms perceived for a long time, or because having MS is experienced as less serious than other diagnoses previously hypothesized (for example, a brain tumor). Appendix 2 contains examples relating to the feelings experienced at the time of diagnosis and expressed through images.

Upon participants having expressed their experiences on these two moments (moment of diagnosis and current moment), the facilitator picks up with what has emerged within the group, focusing attention on various aspects of the described emotions that were present when receiving the diagnosis and those present now. Skillfully, the facilitator interprets the aspects of change that often emerge on an emotional level (usually we move from a greater emotional intensity to a lower and more easily manageable emotionality). This step is due to some individual variables and the time that has passed since the diagnosis was communicated. It is very important to highlight this last element, because within the same group, there may be people who have received the diagnosis a few weeks or a few months ago, and others who have received it for a year or more. The chronological dimension often plays a crucial role in the awareness and processing of the diagnosis and in the emotional changes that follow from that moment on.

During the participants' presentation, the facilitator writes key words and crucial issues on a flipchart, so that she can then summarize the contents that emerged, highlighting the common aspects, peculiarities and differences of each story. After having collected everyone's presentations and proposed a summary, the facilitator asks each participant to answer the question "Who am I?" writing in the appropriate space of their individual file what they consider most salient in relation to this question. The question serves to highlight who you were before the diagnosis and who you are now. The content of what is written on the sheet is not shared with the rest of the group, but remains a personal reflection that can be modified and enriched throughout the course of the intervention.

Finally, participants are advised to perform the fractional breathing exercise independently at home and to read the part of the book *Coping with Chronic Illness. Theories, issues and lived experiences* (Bonino, 2021) in which the topics discussed in the group are addressed, and they meet at the next meeting (for the "homework", here as for all future meetings, see Appendix 1).

The session ends with a relaxation exercise through fractional breathing.

Box 3.2   First meeting: Points and tips for the facilitator

1   Silvia Bonino's introduction is a particular aspect of the groups held at the Cosso Foundation and cannot be carried out in other contexts. However, the group facilitator will be able to use the book *Coping with chronic illness. Theories, issues and lived experiences* (Bonino, 2021) and in particular the preface and the premise *Why this book*, to present the group journey.

2   The inclusion of a positive aspect allows one to start by focusing attention on a resource not affected by the disease. It may happen that some participants say what they liked to do before their illness, but which is no longer possible to do, and it is important to direct the attention of these people to what they still like to do despite MS. This leads the participants

to overcome the narrative of loss and renunciation caused by the disease, in which some people tend to identify with and remain trapped. It may happen that this story brings out strong emotions prematurely in both the speaker and the listener, with consequent discomfort and embarrassment on the part of the participants. In this case, the facilitator must empathically welcome and validate what emerges, monitoring the discomfort and emotional contagion that can spread within the group. This presentation method also allows, on the one hand, to contain those who risk being excessively verbose, and on the other who, due to shyness or otherwise, are hesitant about what to say about themselves. Furthermore, the expressed resource (i.e., a positive aspect of one's life) serves to get to know each other beyond the illness, to arouse curiosity and create interest, starting to weave the process of group union and interaction. When the facilitator perceives rigidity and tension in the group, one of the possible options to dissolve apprehension and facilitate relaxation is a reciprocity exercise. The chosen "icebreaker" game consists in introducing another member of the group by repeating the name and information that one remembers, in particular the resource not affected by the disease. In this way, the memorization not only of the name but also of the characteristics that distinguish that individual is promoted, and if someone does not remember the information, others can intervene to fill the gaps. The result of this collective review is that people begin to interact, smiling when they don't remember some information and thanking them when someone comes to their aid; furthermore, each participant learns the names and characteristics of the others, avoiding spending the entire time of the meeting without remembering and being embarrassed by this. For everyone, then, pleasure is activated in the awareness of feeling recognized in one's individuality. The facilitator can decide to play this game based on the number of participants, the time available and the atmosphere of the moment; it is particularly useful for facilitating ease at work and the creation of a peaceful environment in larger and more rigid groups.

3 The exercise of choosing images, initially not foreseen, was included after having noted that it could be an aid for the participants and a strategy to better manage the following aspects.

- Maintain focus on the request the intervention wants to respond to, that is, the emotional aspect of the illness experience, because participants risk telling their story relating to the period of diagnosis without precisely identifying the feelings that accompanied it.
- Give a name to emotions more easily. It may happen that people are not clear about the distinction between thoughts, emotions and physical sensations; taking up their words when they name emotions helps them to unravel the complexity of what they have felt, or still feel, and to gain clarity within themselves.

- Offer a very specific framework to fit within. This aspect is particularly useful for people who tend to talk more, risking taking away space and time from other participants. If the speaker tends to linger anyway, it will be easier for the facilitator to intervene to bring the narrative exposition back to the delivery.
- Help the more silent or inhibited people, who are helped by the use of the image to direct words onto a concrete object; furthermore, they can keep their gaze on the photo to overcome the initial embarrassment.

In the appendix are some of the images used in the meetings. They represent a hint and a suggestion and can be adapted by the facilitator in relation to individual project contexts.

Second meeting

Box 3.3   Meeting 2 – the restructuring of identity and the search for new objectives capable of giving sense to life

Introduction (1.)

- Fractional breathing
- Previous session review and "homework"
- Introduction of the topics addressed: restructuring of identity, sense of coherence, search for new goals

Contents and topics (2.)

- Explore the following questions in the different life contexts (relationships, work, free time and community)

  a What gave meaning to life before the diagnosis and what gives meaning to one's life now?
  b What could now increase the sense of realization?
  c "Concretely, what could I change to feel that life is worth living, and therefore to live better?"
  d "So who can I be, despite my illness?"

Conclusion (3.)

- Invitation to carry out "homework", see Appendix 1
- Fractional breathing

The restructuring of identity and the search for new objectives capable of giving meaning to life

The group activity begins with the fractional breathing exercise to encourage the acquisition of this practice and resource, to open up a space for discussion and sharing based on body awareness, and, as anticipated, to introduce a practice that becomes a sort of group ritual that marks the beginning of the meeting.

Subsequently, the facilitator asks the participants what they noticed when carrying out the breathing practice at home, leaving space to explain their experience and any doubts or difficulties in carrying out it (see also point 1 of Box 3.4). Attention to how the time between one meeting and another is used is important, and in this first phase, it focuses on practical exercises and their usefulness, regardless of the level of discomfort a person is feeling in the present moment. In fact, these short breaks to be included in one's days are first and foremost a way to take care of oneself, and represent a valid tool for maintaining a high level of perceived well-being where it is already present, while they also represent an optimal way to modulate discomfort, body possibly activated by thoughts, sensations and emotions.

After a brief introduction in which the contents that emerged in the first meeting are summarized, the facilitator introduces the theme of identity restructuring. The objective is to explore what changes, if any, the illness has introduced: specifically, which projects have changed in terms of purpose or timing, and which have possibly been abandoned or suspended. At the same time, we explore what thoughts and emotions accompany this transformation: such as, fear of achieving less? Not having enough time? We will therefore ask ourselves: what does this cause in behavioral terms? An acceleration to be able to do more things, a deceleration or maintaining the plans planned before one's illness without any changes?

The first questions directed to the participants to highlight the changes introduced by the illness on the meaning of one's life are: "How do I see my future with MS, and what changes, if any, has my illness introduced in relation to it?"; "Have my plans changed?"; "Do I think I'm doing things differently?"; "Am I afraid of accomplishing less?"

These points are very important to encourage a good restructuring of identity, understood not as the person's passive remission to the manifestations of their illness, but as a stimulus to assume an active attitude that leads to the identification of both new objectives and the tools and strategies to reach them, thus exercising control over one's life condition. Furthermore, working on the reactivation of one's life plan defuses the arrest "giving in" and the stalemate mechanism that often occurs following the diagnosis of illness. This mechanism represents a suitable emotional reaction when it is directly related to a potentially traumatic event (such as communication of the diagnosis, a relapse of illness, a change in therapy), but it becomes pathological if it persists over time.

The facilitator then directs the reflection on the search for meaning in one's life, signifying with this expression what is important, makes one feel fulfilled and leads one to commit and fight to obtain it. Participants are invited to evaluate what gave meaning before the diagnosis, what gives meaning now and what is possible and useful to change to perceive their life as full of meaning. This reflection is conducted by examining the areas considered most important in life: family, study or work, free time (see also point 2 of Box 3.4).

The topic of objectives and projects that give meaning to life is very delicate and complex. These questions elicit, in general, three possible categories of answers: those who reply that nothing has changed, those who say that everything has changed and nothing makes sense anymore, and those who are amazed by a question that implies meditating on what direction is my life taking.

This last reaction highlights how stopping to think about which guiding principles and priorities motivate and guide one's existence, so that it is lived fully, requires an introspective attitude that is not to be taken for granted. It is therefore normal that this analysis takes time and that there is not necessarily a ready answer to this question.

The immediate statement that the disease has not brought about any changes often hides the profound feeling that MS is in control of one's life. Consequently, the person defensively, completely rejects the idea that the illness could change one's life because such an admission, even partial, would imply the recognition of being entirely subjugated by it. Furthermore, the changes introduced by the disease are often, at this stage, not yet evident from the outside: they consist of new perceptions linked to the self-image and what is important in relationships with others, in one's profession and in free time. In this case, it is useful to underline the importance of noticing even those small changes that illness imposed and which one adapted to, perhaps without too much effort. Often in these cases, it is useful to let the group discussion bring out these aspects, so that the people who deny the change have time to enter into the perspective of the change understood not only as renunciation, but also as the possibility of activating an attitude different, as the possibility of changing behaviors rather than just undergoing changes. This means, therefore, evaluating what, since the advent of one's illness, can still be done despite it, and even more so what may be important to modify to feel that one's life is worth living. The period following the diagnosis is crucial for working on the connection with one's desires and projects, precisely because one can systematize any changes that have already been implemented, and evaluate those that can be made now to improve one's quality of life.

Those who claim that MS has changed everything, experience the disease as an omnipotent reality, which has become the absolute protagonist of their thoughts, emotions and sensations experienced. The help, in this case, is aimed at reducing the space that MS occupies in the people's life, so that they open up to new projects. Reflection on the current objectives that give meaning to life, and which at the same time favor the development of future projects, therefore serves to promote an active and proactive attitude, implicitly going to undermine the patterns of total rupture and contrast between life before illness, full of possibilities, and that after the diagnosis, in which everything takes on the meaning of loss and surrender. Also in this case, comparison with other members of the group can encourage the emergence of aspects that can be usefully explored together with other people who feel trapped by the disease (see the examples given in Appendix 2).

In this regard, let's go back to the progress of the meeting. During the explanation of the contents, the facilitator notes the themes that emerge on the flip chart so that it is also easy for the participants who are listening to pick up on the content and make a connection with their own experience. Furthermore, these notes become the tool with which the final summary and re-elaboration of the contents will be built, with which we will continue to work in subsequent meetings. In fact, the material that emerges is "dynamic" material, that is, evolving, because these reflections presuppose the activation of an increasingly greater awareness of oneself, of one's objectives, of resources that can facilitate the achievement of these goals and the limits that must be faced.

During the meetings, the theme of limits is a constant that sometimes goes unnoticed, but which is always useful to explain. Often when we think about the limitations linked to MS we immediately imagine the difficulties associated with walking and the consequent use of aids such as crutches, walkers and wheelchairs. As already mentioned, this vision, which activates worrying thoughts and disturbing emotions, is the first image that is generally associated with this illness. In reality, we know that the limitations that this illness imposes are not necessarily linked to walking, but have to do with other aspects related to the body, with other symptoms, and with the relationship that everyone establishes with these. In fact, if on the one hand, the symptom makes an objective limit manifesting (deficit in strength, difficulty in fine movements, bladder disorders, fatigue, etc.), on the other hand, each person relates to this limit in a subjective way, through adaptive reactions and the development of effective strategies, or vice versa through non-adaptive reactions and ineffective strategies. Consequently, it is important that the person activates an adaptation process, on a psychological level, centered on the change imposed by MS, in which flexibility, the willingness to welcome, integrate and therefore accept these changes becomes an evolutionary constant. Obviously, this process occurs over time, and it is likely that those who have received the diagnosis longer have developed greater awareness, while those who have been diagnosed more recently are still in a phase of disorientation and confusion, perceptible on a cognitive, emotional and physical level. So, on the one hand, for those who have been living with the disease for longer, talking about the limits, and evaluating what adjustments can be made in light of this new presence, becomes a way to systematize the skills acquired with respect to symptom management. On the other hand, for those who have had MS for a shorter time, talking about it is a support and a useful help to explore their experiences, increasing awareness of their experiences and what happens in the body, in less time than necessary to people who do not have the opportunity to interact in a group with others. Also for this aspect, group discussion is an incomparable resource.

The group facilitator therefore has the task of stimulating people to work together, in the group, on the restructuring of identity, redefining the aspects of the latter that have been modified by the illness.

In particular, it is important to help those people who are locked in following the image of themselves before the diagnosis, thus risking falling into the psychological traps linked to the continuous use of illusory thinking ("Nothing has changed") or negative thinking ("I've lost everything") and activating dysfunctional behaviors that inhibit the creation of a new identity structure.

In addition to collecting the information that comes from the participants and re-elaborating upon it together, the facilitator also clarifies some often unconscious psychological mechanisms that favor or negatively influence a good adaptation to their illness. For example, the facilitator explains that to build a "healthy" and "balanced" relationship with the limits imposed by this illness, it is necessary to move away from the idea of challenge, understood as the need to ignore these limits and go beyond them: often, in the current culture which pushes us to over-come every limit, this idea is triggered automatically. Confronting a limit of MS means understanding how far you can push yourself on a physical level and when it is necessary to stop to avoid dangerous consequences. This involves learning to listen to the body and self-observation, noticing what the effects of limits are and what adjustments can be made to grow from them. Even more, if the concept of challenge activates the vision of attack toward something that is attacking, and that something is one's own body, then it is clear that fighting against one's illness becomes a dangerous way of relating to oneself. The idea promoted in the group is taking care of oneself, of one's body and therefore of one's illness, being able to listen to its limits and implementing procedures to avoid worsening one's physical condition, but rather consistently remaining proactive, yet very respectful of what the body may or may not do any longer.

The concrete ways to effectively address this aspect, as well as to achieve new objectives capable of giving meaning to one's life, will be examined in the third meeting.

The second meeting ends with the invitation to rethink the contents that emerged in the group through the outline of the meeting and to dedicate oneself to the other "homework" (see Appendix 1), followed by the relaxation exercise through frac-tional breathing.

Box 3.4   Second meeting: Points and tips for the facilitator

1 Checking that participants have taken the time to carry out the practice at home is essential, as it serves to create a space dedicated to themselves within their daily lives. It is important to take care of this aspect initially, to encourage the use of the breathing exercise, and thus make it truly en-ter the "toolbox" of each participant. Subsequently, or sometimes already starting from this second meeting, it will be the participants themselves who will describe the contexts in which they have applied fractional breathing and who will describe how this has positively influenced the in-crease in psycho-emotional balance and therefore on their own well-being.

2 It is useful to reassure people that all of us, in general, rarely stop at this type of reflection, and that being able to do so in group helps to put

thoughts into circulation and evaluate deeply what is important to us. It can be underlined how these questions should be left to settle to evaluate what effects it produces not only at that moment, but also over time, and therefore after that the topic was developed in a group (it is in fact very likely that thoughts emerge about it even after the meeting).

Third meeting

Box 3.5   Meeting 3 – self-efficacy in achieving one's objectives and in managing their symptoms

Introduction (1.)

- Fractional breathing
- Previous session review and "homework"
- Introduction of the themes addressed: restructuring of identity, self-efficacy, symptom management

Contents and topics (2.)

- Reading, in-depth analysis and comparison on the handout provided
- Ask which of the suggestions contained in the handout one already follows, then choose one or more new ones to introduce into the own daily life
- Define which objectives are significant but obtainable at the same time, possibly changing them in various areas of life (relationships, work, free time)
- Identify precise strategies (modalities, steps, help from others) to achieve these objectives. In particular, predict the difficulties and how they can be done overcome
- Evaluate your own behavior, both in case of success and failure, and make any necessary adjustments

Conclusion (3.)

- Invitation to carry out "homework", see Appendix 1
- Fractional breathing

Self-efficacy in achieving goals and managing symptoms

This meeting opens, as the others, with the relaxation exercise through fractional breathing. When finished, the facilitator picks up the theme introduced during the previous meeting (what can give meaning to life and make one feel fulfilled and satisfied?) connecting it to the current topic of: self-efficacy in achieving objectives and managing symptoms.

Participants are explained that to engage in significant actions, to achieve important and precise objectives, one needs to be sure that they have the necessary resources to face such actions and to carry them to completion. Consequently, finding meaning in one's life and concretizing it in an identity that is committed to achieving specific objectives, requires a good feeling of self-efficacy, that is, the sense of security given by being aware of how to face a situation and how to achieve what one has proposed: having the resources, or knowing where to find them, and knowing how to do it, what strategies to use, what steps to follow. In this way, one feels they have control over situations and their lives.

Due to one's illness, all this is in serious crisis. Even if it is not possible to control the illness, which has no definitive cure, it is however possible to regain control over everyday life, which passes, above all, from the awareness of knowing how to correctly manage physical and emotional disorders.

To explore and develop this last point, the facilitator focuses the discussion on strategies to better manage fatigue, a very common symptom that has a strong impact on the person's quality of life. The topic is addressed accordingly self-observation, a method that allows for greater awareness of one's internal experiences, both physical and emotional, and an effective tool for mapping one's sensations.

Through self-observation, a way of paying attention to oneself is introduced which is often dysregulated, especially at the beginning of the illness. In fact, the subject suddenly experiences new and anomalous physical sensations in their own body (for example, paresthesia, diplopia, paralysis of a limb or half of the body), which inevitably frightens one. This fear activates the limbic system at the brain level, producing automatic responses of alarm and hypervigilance. Consequently, the person is very attentive to what they perceive and is very attentive in grasping every sensation; however, due to the hyperactivation of the internal alarm system, there is a risk of interpreting physical sensations and signs as symptoms of illness which are not (see point 1 of Box 3.6). It may happen, therefore, that the interpretation of what the individual feels is distorted by the erroneous activation of the internal alarm system, which evaluates as "dangerous" elements that in reality they are not. Furthermore, fear and anxiety can contribute to increasing the perception of that sensation, consequently amplifying the discomfort.

It should be emphasized that some people try to use avoidance as a tool to not feel, to not take into account what the body feels. But we know that, in addition to being extremely tiring, it is certainly very unuseful and ineffective to alienate oneself from one's body and pretend that it has no reactions. Sometimes, however, this dysfunctional strategy finds support in the words of some healthcare professionals who advise the patient "not to listen to the body too much". The result is that the person hears a lot, but chooses to listen little. If trust and security in one's body are already profoundly undermined by their illness, the attitude of indifference to what the body experiences fuels a maladaptive defensive mode. Conscious self-observation instead allows for greater familiarity with the symptoms and emotional regulation that allow us to understand what may indicate an attack or worsening of the illness and what is nothing more than a fluctuation of symptoms.

To become more familiar with the symptoms and improve one's ability to understand the manifestations of the disease, the facilitator reads aloud from the paper material that is distributed to the participants (Appendix 1, third meeting), starting with the rules for improving fatigue management and optimizing energy savings. The instructions given to the participants are to mentally note down if among these there are any measures that they already use, and if there are any suggestions that can be introduced into one's daily life to further improve one's energy management ability.

Following then, the group work passes from a mode of private and personal reflection on one's history of illness to a more concrete and timely evaluation of the individual elements that can positively or negatively influence the well-being of each individual person. Each participant is therefore asked, by telling the group the strategies they already use in their everyday experience, and also to establish if and how they are implementing the principles of energy saving and symptom management. We therefore give systematicity and value to the skills already learned in the field, activating a virtuous circle in which each person tells how they introduced a change into their life and what positive effects it has had. This comparison and sharing of experiences facilitate self-observation in everyone, even in those who are less accustomed to reflecting on their own experiences. By listening to other persons and how they have put that particular strategy into practice in their daily lives, participants can make comparisons and establish whether they have also implemented this adaptation in their own lives, and in what way have they inserted it, or perhaps they haven't had need to. People who have received the diagnosis shortly before are in an orientation phase, and therefore do not yet have a sufficiently structured experience to draw conclusions about symptom management. However, they can equally benefit from this group work. In fact, if on the one hand their intervention will be reduced, on the other they will be provided with a wide range of possible strategies in case those difficulties arise. It's like having a large and specific toolbox to counteract any problems that may arise in the future.

In structuring the meeting, the next question asks the participants to explain their personal objectives: they will evaluate what the important and sustainable goals may be, in terms of realistic expectations adhering to the current situation (see point 2 of Box 3.6). The question is therefore: "What goals are or could be important and significant for me, but at the same time achievable (possibly changing the ones I had)?".

The areas explored are primarily emotional relationships and the family. We then review the purposes inherent in friendship relationships, work and free time.

The objectives are the concretization, in terms of actions, of what was defined in the second meeting as a value that is significant – giving a sense of fulfillment to life. This outlines the direction we undertake or maintain, like a lighthouse that orients the navigator to keep the course steady while addressing possible dangers, such as reefs or shallows.

Once the objectives expressed by the group members have been identified, the facilitator writes the question on the flipchart: "What precise strategies can allow me to achieve the set objective?".

Therefore, it is not enough to identify objectives: it is also necessary to be clear which steps, aids, and resources can be put in place as strategies to achieve the desired goal.

The reflection process ends with a further question, relating to the final evaluation of the result and the strategies used. If, according to the evaluation, the objective has been achieved, the behavior adopted in that case will be maintained, otherwise each person will have to appeal to their cognitive and action flexibility to make the adjustments necessary to achieve their goals. This question, which reads: "How can I evaluate my behavior and make the necessary adjustments?", is then also written on the flip chart, so that the three phases of the process of strengthening self-efficacy are clearly visible: definition of objectives (first question); choice of possible useful strategies to achieve the goal (second question); evaluation of the result and redefinition of the tools, if those used were not sufficiently effective (third question).

The meeting ends with the breathing exercise, which follows the request to carry out the "homework" and to let what has emerged during the time spent together settle, noting any reflections and new elements that come out as a result of the work done together.

The material that was shared with the group is a dynamic material, "in movement", so some aspects often need a time to mature, in the interiority of the individual, like seeds that are planted and that need some time to express themselves. Furthermore, the process of change is in itself a transformative evolution, which undoubtedly needs time to be implemented and maintained.

Box 3.6   Third meeting: Points and tips for the facilitator

1 Based on the information about symptoms, neurologists provide when explaining in which cases to go to hospital for an urgent visit, seems easy discriminate what is a symptom. In fact, doctors define the presence of a new attack of the disease as the appearance of new symptoms, or the worsening of existing symptoms, for a duration of 24 hours, in

the absence of fever and infections, and if at least one month has passed since the previous attack. The unconscious activation of assiduous internal monitoring, which looks anxiously at everything that is experienced, but it often makes it difficult, in practice, to discriminate whether what you feel is a "normal" bodily experience, or an exacerbation due to the disease, and therefore a neurological symptom.

2 The goal of returning to how we were before the illness in physical terms it is not an achievable goal. Of course sometimes, it happens that following a relapse of the disease the symptoms may regress and disappear completely, but these are sporadic cases. Furthermore, awareness remains that there is a chronic disease that, if it does not manifest itself explicitly – with signs and symptoms, it is still present in the body due to lesions in the myelin sheath.

Fourth meeting

Box 3.7   Meeting 4 – emotions, sensations and thoughts

Introduction (1.)

- Fractional breathing
- Previous session review and "homework"

Contents and topics (2.)

- Topics addressed: thought and emotions management
- Reading, in-depth study and comparison on the material of handout
- Ask which of the suggestions contained in the handout one already follows, then choose one or more new ones to introduce into the own daily life

Conclusion (3.)

- Invitation to carry out "homework", see Appendix 1
- Fractional breathing, stabilization and centering of self

Emotions, sensations and thoughts

The group meeting opens, as the others, with the relaxation exercise through fractional breathing. The facilitator then returns to the theme to which the previous meeting was dedicated, namely, the effective realization of one's objectives, to recover or give a new meaning to one's life, while at the same time also rediscovering a sense of control over oneself and about daily life.

The reactivation of a sense of control is linked to the ability to know how to manage emotions, so as not to be overwhelmed by them even when they are very intense, and therefore not to implement avoidance mechanisms that do nothing but increase emotional pressure.

This introduces the theme to which we will dedicate ourselves in the meeting: the link between emotions, thoughts and physical sensations. The facilitator highlights how this link can influence a self-reinforcing vicious circle, exacerbating a spiral of negative emotions, sensations and thoughts, or on the contrary favor a spiral that promotes positive circularity.

The first part of the meeting is therefore dedicated to the explanation of the structural and conjunction mechanisms of thoughts, emotions and physical sensations, which are closely interconnected. Through the material called *Positive and Negative Circularity* (found in Appendix 1), the facilitator delves into the dynamics that are established when a worrying or negative thought emerges – which activates emotions such as anxiety, sadness, fear, anger – and how these resonate in the body through physical sensations considered unpleasant (see point 1 of Box 3.8). These three elements (thoughts, emotions, physical sensations) are the expression of internal states that can be dominated by the dysregulation of the autonomic nervous system, which, in this case, instead of being balanced between the two systems that compose it (system orthosympathetic and parasympathetic), it is hyper-activated in the direction of one or the other, resulting in fight/flight or block/submission reactions. The results of the excess activation of one or another system are the basis of our non-adaptive behaviors, and in this negative spiral, the actions implemented will be dysfunctional and not suitable for achieving the goals one has set for themselves. Conversely, in positive circularity, characterized by neutral or positive thoughts and congruent emotions and physical sensations, the actions we activate will be suitable for our purposes and this will favor the reinforcement of that circuit.

Participants are explained how it is possible to intervene on each element of the circuit to favor the exit from the negative circularity and the entry into the positive one, or to remain within the positive one. In fact, it is possible to intervene on thoughts (from top to bottom or top-down) through self-observation and awareness of the power of our cognitions to desensitize and reprocess strong emotions that produce physical sensations that are difficult to manage. At the same time, however, it is possible to choose another path, and use a "bottom-up" intervention, i.e., an intervention that starts from the body with its emotional and physical manifestations, and modulate these elements by eliciting a secondary effect on thoughts, which will subsequently be perceived as less disturbing.

Once the circuit has been explained and how we all function, it is important to pause, and ask participants if they have concrete examples to share with the group. In this way, it is possible to verify that the understanding of the "circle" has actually occurred, and above all that it is clear what emotions are, what thoughts are and what physical sensations are. Experience has taught us that people often believe they know what emotions are but in fact recognize few of them, often confusing them and mistaking them for physical sensations (see point 2 of Box 3.8). Through the activity of sharing concrete experiences, participants increase their emotional vocabulary and their way of relating to physical sensations. This is possible thanks to the activation of an attentive and focused attitude on what you feel in your body and where you feel it. In trying to be as precise as possible, we will not do so in an obsessive manner, but with the aim of noticing the details of our perceptions, focusing on a deeper and unfleeting listening. This approach has a double advantage: first of all, it favors the connection with internal perceptions, which are listened to rather than avoided, shunned, or suppressed. As previously anticipated, these latter methods are ineffective; in fact, if in an initial moment of avoidance and escape from one's own perceptions, it appears the body returns to a sensorial silence, subsequently the emotion and sensation physical effects will be even more intense and the person will therefore experience an even greater sense of loss of control. Familiarizing yourself with what you feel in your body means feeling less afraid, and therefore choosing to connect with your internal experiences. This internal observer position represents the second advantage, since it involves feeling that you can manage what you feel, and therefore also increasing one's self-efficacy.

Having analyzed this circularity providing an understanding of which mechanisms at a psycho-physical level it triggers, the meeting continues with an in-depth analysis of every single element that constitutes the vicious circle, in the case of a negative trigger, or virtuous one, in the case of a positive trigger.

The material *From thought to emotions: thoughts can increase or reduce stress* (see Appendix 1 and point 3 of Box 3.8) divides thoughts into the categories of "positive", "negative" and "illusory": the facilitator asks for three volunteers who are then asked to impersonate the three types of thoughts by reading the proposed examples aloud. They are examples of how the same event can be interpreted differently based on the type of cognitive filter that the person is applying and which leads to thinking about the event in a positive, negative or illusory way.

The opening questions after reading the sentences are: "Where do you place yourself in relation to these types of thinking?"; "What type of thought do you lean toward with respect to the three proposed?". Everyone thus has the opportunity to stop and reflect on what type of reading of reality they tend to make. It spontaneously emerges that negative thinking is easily distinguishable. People often verbalize that they have had periods in which they've experienced the lens of negative thinking and what happened to them, but then they realize they had changed their vision, moving toward a more positive one. Some participants, however, say they tend toward negative thoughts, while someone else feels more represented by the other two types of thinking. It is at this moment that the facilitator emphasizes the importance of recognizing the frequency with which one uses a certain type of thought. In fact, negative thinking is not to be demonized: it is normal and physiological for an event that creates discomfort and suffering is accompanied by a negative thought. However, the important aspect is to evaluate how the use of this type of thinking is temporary and closely linked to certain occurrences that happen, or how much it is a constant way of reading reality. It is in this second case that it is important to intervene modifying this tendency by encouraging the activation of positive thoughts.

A second element to call attention to is the "structure" of positive thinking. A further opening question submitted to the group is: "What do you notice in positive thinking? What characteristics does it have?". The aim of this question is to single out the fact that positive thinking starts from the awareness of what has happened; it is not a denial of what happened, its devaluation, trivialization or, even worse, the sarcasm that one can use to escape the vicious circle of negative thinking. This reflection is critically important, because easily people can have a distorted vision of what "positive thinking" means.

Positive thinking is often associated with the mistaken idea that it is enough to want something, to be sufficiently motivated, for it to happen. But this easy access slogan represents a heuristic that does not take into account the complexity of the psyche. In fact, the term "positivity" does not simplistically mean thinking and saying positive things despite one feeling something completely different. To implement significant changes in the medium and long terms, there is no need to "cover" the experiences endured with positive words, denying the underlying physical sensations and emotions, and it is counterproductive to adopt a denialist mental attitude in which a mantra constructed with positive words is mechanically repeated.

It needs to be explained that it is necessary to defuse the automatic pilot of the fictitious and superficial use of positive thinking, to instead invest in a more optimistic and self-confident attitude and in one's ability to deal with experiences. Initially, this process of change will involve an effort, but subsequently it will become a natural and spontaneous way of approaching events.

Positive thinking therefore starts from the observation of what happened and shifts attention to what can be done, despite an alarming, tense experience. If we translate positive thinking to the experiences of illness, we can say that it consists of a cognitive approach in which the limits imposed by MS are evaluated and, it's from this point, we turn our attention to the analysis of residual potential (see point 4 of Box 3.8).

Another point to pay attention to is the distinction between positive and illusory thinking. Before explaining their dissimilarities, the group is asked the explicit question: "In your opinion, what difference is there between these two types of thinking? What do you notice?". In this way, it emerges whether people actually grasp the subtle distinction between one modality and another. Furthermore, the interaction with the participants increases the possibility of detecting who uses this cognitive scheme because they identify with it, and they can consequently express how and when they use illusory thinking.

The next step is to accompany the group toward understanding what mechanism lies behind the illusory thoughts, i.e., the denial of the problem with the consequent implementation of dysfunctional and non-constructive actions with respect to adaptation. It may happen that the automatic, falsely positive response to negative and intrusive thoughts regarding the illness is replaced by the use of illusory thoughts, which diminishes the emotional experience and gives a false perception of control over one's life. These thoughts are based on non-acceptance and lead to the impossibility of integrating the illness into one's life in a conscious and balanced way. This balance is characterized, on the one hand, by giving space to one's illness, the limits it imposes and the difficulties it presents, but without identifying completely and exclusively with it. On the other hand, it implies leaving space for all aspects of life, not just those that involve managing the disease, to direct one's energies toward what makes one feel good and makes one feel fulfilled.

Illusory thinking is particularly subtle in the context of an illness such as MS, because it can happen that, for even relatively long periods of time, a person feels well, has no disturbing symptoms to deal with, has no relapses, the progression is slow and recognizable only after the passage of time. In this particular context, illusory thinking leads the person to encounter some mental traps and distorted perceptions, such as believing themselves capable of optimally managing their illness and the emotions linked to it. However, when the disease manifests itself again, through a relapse or all the other possible modalities, the individual will inevitably have to confront reality, with one's own way of being, with the aggravating circumstance of not having made any progress in terms of re-elaboration and acceptance of one's condition; the path will therefore be even more tiring and painful than for those who have instead triggered a process of acceptance and adaptation to their illness.

The reading of the handout provided regarding the three types of thoughts ends with the indication to note, as "homework" for the two weeks following the meeting: first of all, which type of thoughts each person tends to engage in and second, how the use of negative or illusory cognition could be modified by activating a positive mode.

The following contribution in Appendix 1 is entitled *Small rules to manage emotions that are a source of suffering and encourage positive ones* and is a list of good practices that everyone can implement to increase their window of emotional tolerance. These are cognitive strategies that help activate coping issues, and the tools to listen to your body and have a greater awareness of one's way of being in terms of physical sensations and emotions.

In closing, after having reminded all to dedicate themselves to their "homework", we renew fractional breathing with insight into the light of the meeting we have just had. Specifically, lengthening the time dedicated to the initial part of listening to the contact points of the body resting on the surfaces that support it, increasing the sense of rootedness and stabilization (see point 5 of Box 3.8). Thereafter, time is left to listen and feel the emotions and sensations that flow in the body, to increase individual awareness of what one's sensing. Finally, the facilitator guides attention to the breath, to the air entering and the air exiting, welcoming the breath as it is without modifying it. This aspect is also important in order to give time to listen and feel the breath, noting where it is felt most (at the level of the nostrils, in the throat, on the chest or in the abdomen; see also point 6 of Box 3.8). After a few breaths, the facilitator introduces the splitting of the inhalation.

The meeting ends with a request for feedback on the sensations felt during the breathing exercise by all participants, and an appointment is made two weeks later for the last meeting of the two-week cycle.

Box 3.8   Fourth meeting: Points and tips for the facilitator

1   It is essential to explain that the goal is not to not feel certain emotions, but *being able to manage them*. In fact, people often have erroneous ideas on how to manage emotions and above all judgmental conceptions of what is correct or mistaken to feel. This judgment assumes that there are emotions that give pleasant sensations and therefore right, and emotions that elicit unpleasant sensations and therefore to be avoided. Instead, we need to educate ourselves to welcome all types of emotion, explaining that it is physiological that the entire emotional range that we have at our disposal can be perceived. Let's therefore pay attention not only to whether a certain emotion is present or not, but with what intensity it manifests itself.

2   It is always useful to underline the *distinction between physical and emotional sensations*. In our experience, it is good to mention both the main emotions (such as fear, anger, sadness) as well as the range of possible physical sensations associated with them (e.g., lump in the throat, weight/tightness in the chest, stomach burning/punching).

3   Often the onset of the disease is associated with a stressful life event, and this leads many to mentally create a connection almost causal between the appearance of MS and stress. In this regard, it is important to clarify that to date the numerous studies carried out in this field have concluded that there is insufficient evidence to argue that stress is a cause of the manifestation of illness (Briones-Buixassa et al., 2015). However, the opposite is true: the factors linked to MS (symptoms, therapies, unpredictability and chronic specificity of the pathology, thoughts and emotions associated with it) can cause great stress. It is worth clarifying this point to give the right role for stress and to explain what is meant by the title of contribution of Appendix 1 *From thought to emotions: thought can increase or reduce stress*. It should therefore be made clear that stress is not the cause of the disease, and it is living in the illusion of controlling all the possible sources of stress with which one comes into contact risks being an ineffective, self-defeating and itself a cause of great stress.

4   In the context of illness, the positive approach responds to the phrase: "Despite MS I can…". Use this mode with the participants, it is useful because it represents group training where everyone can express a positive way of thinking.

5   We are at the fourth meeting and the participants have now done it several times this exercise, so it is possible to deepen the experience by increasing the time dedicated to listening to the breath to work more deeply on

awareness. Here, there is increasing emphasis on listening and feeling without having to do anything except stay in touch with what happens, moment after moment. So the proposed *modality is based on being rather than doing*, experiencing the present through the ability to anchor attention on one stimulus and to be able to intentionally move from one stimulus to another. Self-regulation of attention, and focused awareness on the non-judgmental observation of experience in the here and now, being critical components of *mindfulness* practice. Mindfulness is now widely studied in scientific literature and recognized as a tool to achieve a better inner balance.

6 It is very useful to underline that the invitation is to feel breath and not to think. It might seem trivial, but in reality, if people are not used to this type of listening, they risk activating thought and not focusing their attention on what they feel. To facilitate this observation, a list of possibilities may be suggested: for example, feeling if the breathing is long, short, deep, shallow, labored or regular.

Fifth meeting

Box 3.9   Meeting 5 – communication

Introduction (1.)

- Fractional breathing
- Previous session review and "homework"

Contents and topics (2.)

- Topics addressed: management of communication
- Reading, in-depth study and comparison on the material of handout provided
- Ask which of the suggestions contained in the handout one already follows, then choose one or more new one to introduce into the own daily life

Conclusion (3.)

- Invitation to carry out "homework", see Appendix 1
- Compilation of the questionnaire *Me and my life*
- Compilation of the satisfaction questionnaire *My point of view*
- Fractional breathing, stabilization and centering of self

Communication

After the practice of fractional breathing, the meeting dedicated to communicating with others and asking for help begins.

In fact, it is a theme that emerges throughout the group journey and is therefore addressed indirectly also in previous meetings. Particularly in the first meeting, when people describe their reaction to the diagnosis, they inevitably also refer to the people close to them. This opens up the analysis and problematization of how communicating the diagnosis of MS to other people can be synonymous with help and emotional support from others, but often also with difficulties, because the latter can also develop worrying thoughts and distressing emotional experiences that are added to those of the patient.

In the introductory part, the facilitator therefore takes up what emerged in the first meeting with respect to the choices that everyone made regarding the communication of the diagnosis: to whom it was communicated in the family, friend or work context, when and for what purpose. For some, the need was to tell everyone of their diagnosis, because it is difficult to keep the news to oneself. This automatic communication is probably a way to become aware of the new reality of having a chronic illness. So saying it to others also means repeating it to yourself at the same time. Someone else, however, may be initially very reticent and doesn't want to tell anyone, or is unable to talk to people for fear that by mentioning their illness they will then be invaded by related emotions.

These automatic ways of reacting to the advent of the disease are found not only in patients but also in people close to them, especially family members. Sometimes, it happens that the latter confides in other relatives or friends in order to share the burden of the situation. This sharing is not always agreed upon with the person with MS and this can also generate heated conflicts. This is the first aspect linked to communication dynamics.

The second aspect, addressed in the meeting concerns communicating effectively with others, an indispensable strategy for feeling good and succeeding to achieve the objectives that are considered important in all sectors of life, also thanks to the help of others.

But to ask for help from others one must first be willing to receive help. Others can be a useful support only if there is a willingness to open up and accept another's help. It therefore becomes essential to reflect and have a clear understanding of one's internal position regarding receiving help. Often the people we meet in groups have a distorted vision of asking for help, associating the request with being weak or not independent. Independence is a fundamental aspect for people with MS, and it is important to be able to maintain and decline it in one's life based on the characteristics of the illness. However, stubbornly persevering in doing everything alone, to avoid asking for support from others is a rigid and defensive attitude, not beneficial to achieving one's goals.

Just as being ill does not mean having to rely on others, it does not mean the exact opposite either. It is therefore important to convey the message of normalization of the request for help, which must be seen as a possibility that can positively influence the achievement of one's objectives.

In fact, communicating well with others also serves to ask them for help in the correct way: neither too much nor too little, and at the right time (these elements are detailed in the contribution in Appendix 1 *Learning to ask others for help (family, friends, colleagues)*; also see point 1 of Box 3.10).

Reference is made here to two other important aspects: one's own value and the dimension of reciprocity.

In regard to the first aspect, the focus is on self-perception in relation to the request for help. If one's individual value is linked to a dysfunctional cognition for which asking for support means decreasing self-esteem and belittling one's qualities, then it is obvious that it will be difficult to request it (see point 2 of Box 3.10). Furthermore, emotions such as shame, embarrassment, guilt, anxiety or fear of expressing a need can intervene, which also inhibits communication with others. Instead, it becomes fundamental to insist on the possibility of creating a fruitful dialogue with others in order to proceed day by day toward a greater understanding of MS and its mechanisms within one's specific context.

The dimension of reciprocity, i.e., the possibility of being able to return the help received in some way, is an aspect generally rarely taken into consideration by the participants, which opens up the possibility of not feeling indebted or unequal to another. Consequently, it helps to convey a positive self-image, as a person capable of taking care of the needs of others, and not as merely needy because they are ill. Although this aspect is rationally easily understandable and clear, in reality people may tend not to think of themselves as possible supports and help for others, especially at the beginning of the disease or when MS makes itself particularly felt with the limitations it imposes.

Another important element to reflect on is the variations of challenges related to managing certain symptoms. Especially at the beginning, the newly diagnosed person must learn to take "measures" of the symptomatic manifestations. For example, fatigue often presents fluctuations of intensity, meaning sometimes it is possible to do certain activities, even demanding ones from an energetic point of view, which at other times are impossible to complete. When there is an irregularity in the presentation of symptoms, it is difficult to be able to describe and make others understand such fluctuating manifestations.

The material in Appendix 1 *Rules of good communication with others (family, friends, colleagues)* particularly focuses on what is not said and what can happen. One of the errors in communication is relying on the idea that others understand what we want without making it explicit: since everything seems so obvious and clear to us, we think that it is perceivable in the same way for others too. The fact that others do not respond to our unexpressed expectations activates an inhibition circuit that becomes increasingly stronger, in a sort of negative circularity of communication based on the thought "I don't ask, because they don't understand or it's useless anyway". So the first step is to express one's need without waiting for others to guess or notice what is desired but kept silent. The second aspect, closely linked to the first, is to avoid malicious interpretations of why others do not guess whether help is needed or not, hence they do not offer it. Finally, once it is clear in one's mind what you need, without assuming that what is clear and crystalline for us is also clear for others, you must verbalize the sentence in a precise and clear way. Many misunderstandings are the result of communications that did not take place, or of communications occurred partially or with ambiguous formulations, which do not take into account that everyone's conceptual map is different; the risk that the message does not reach the recipient, or that a partial or even different message compared to the one intended to be conveyed, is very high (see point 3 of Box 3.10).

In the *Rules of self-observation,* a brief idea which is found, like the previous ones, in the materials relating to the fifth meeting of Appendix 1, the focus of attention returns exclusively to oneself, with the aim of clarifying first and foremost to oneself, and as much as possible, the progress of the symptoms and noticing what happens to the body, in order to acquire more and more awareness and familiarity with what one feels. This is an indispensable premise for having a clear idea of how to respond to doctors during visits, and what to ask when one has doubts or needs further explanations regarding the illness and its manifestations in one's body (see also point 4 of Box 3.10).

Finally, in the *Rules of communication with healthcare professionals,* the last of the materials of the fifth meeting (Appendix 1), the salient aspects to be taken into consideration every time neurological visits are carried out are explained. Through the first point, we want to legitimize the patient to request explanations in case one has doubts or does not understand something. It seems obvious, but often people, out of shame, fear or anxiety of being judged by the doctor, prefer to pretend to have grasped concepts and information that in reality they have not understood and consequently not even learned. The medical visit is a moment shared between the healthcare staff and the patient in which there must be the necessary time to visit, ask questions and receive answers. It is no longer conceivable that communication occurs one way, from the "active" doctor, who speaks, to the "passive" patient, who just listens, as was taken for granted in the past. It is now well established that good communication is an act of cooperation in which shared meanings are built, in a bidirectional and not unidirectional relationship. This is even more true in the therapeutic action. The professional is the facilitator of the interview, and as such, gives space and time to the other to be able to process the information given, allowing for an expression of what one feels is important in relation to the aspects addressed in the sharing of their meanings.

In the second point of the *Rules of communication with healthcare professionals,* it is recommended to ask healthcare professionals to write down all the instructions given relating to therapy and drug management. In fact, not only is every communicative interaction subject to filters, but also the steps between understanding the information received, its storage and its actual use lead to the inevitable loss of data; consequently, it is essential to have a written text.

For the same reasons, it is also useful to write down the instructions yourself, as suggested to do for your own emotions (Appendix 1, Fourth meeting, *Small rules to manage emotions that are sources of suffering and encourage positive ones*). For example, the moment when the nursing staff teaches a newly diagnosed person – proposes as a first therapeutic option, one of the drugs commonly referred to as "first-line" – how and when to inject, in which points of the body, how to prevent and manage any side effects, is an excellent circumstance to write down the strategies and advice given. All the useful information regarding taking the therapy is written on the drug information leaflet. However, having specialized personnel at your disposal who teach and demonstrate how to carry out the injection and having the opportunity to ask questions and resolve any doubts by noting down the answers is a precious added value that fuels the sense of self-efficacy with respect to drug management. This aspect is developed in the third point of the *Rules of communication with healthcare professionals.*

Having reached this point, the facilitator concludes the part of the intervention dedicated to the theme of communication and opens a space dedicated to retracing all the meetings in salient points. This summary serves to "refresh" the topics discussed and allow everything that emerged during the meetings to settle (see also point 5 of Box 3.10).

You are finally reminded to do your "homework".

Following, the *Me and my life* questionnaire (Appendix 4) is again administered to the participants together with a short evaluation sheet of the path taken called *My point of view* (Appendix 5).

The group ends with the practice of breathing awareness and the facilitator reminds us that we will see each other again in about six months.

Box 3.10   Fifth meeting: Points and tips for the facilitator

1 After reading the points contained in this contribution, it is useful to stop and give the group space to give concrete examples of what is to come suggested, to bring these aspects into the reality of each one. In particular, in relation to the first point, it may happen that someone argues that people should understand what the ill person needs without having to explicitly verbalize it. Instead, explain that clarity leads to a decrease in misunderstandings and frustrating experiences is important to activate the effort necessary to improve one's communication.

2 This thought is often not expressed openly, but it remains under track. Instead, it is useful to bring it out so that we can talk about it, to interrupt the distorted association between the need for help and decrease in the value attributed to oneself.

3 This aspect highlights the responsibility of communication, which must be understood in its bidirectional nature; the trend, supported by feelings of anger and frustration, it may be to give everything responsibility for ineffective communication to others. This intake can lead to even more frustration, because we feel and think of ourselves as powerless, withholding communication with others something beyond one's control. The result is a passive and defeatist, non-collaborative attitude. The communication is instead an act of collaboration (Grice, 1989). More specifically, on communication in the therapeutic relationship (see Solari et al., 2007; Thompson et al., 2022).

4   This is a very delicate point, since it can happen that the message conveyed by health workers is not to give too much importance to the body, citing the risk of incorrectly interpreting the signals. Indeed, the person may think that those whom they notice are the signs and symptoms of a relapse when in fact they are just fluctuations of the symptoms. *Definitely, an obsessive attitude toward one's own body is not a useful way to deal with the disease, but it is important that the message does not go too far in the opposite direction, and does not cause a failure to listen to or denial of bodily perceptions.* Indeed, inhibiting bodily experiences that make their way with arrogance, not only is it extremely difficult, but it is also extremely harmful, because an individual learns that there is no need to give space to the body and, consequently, one learns not to listen to it, in the illusion of being able to silence and anesthetize.

5   Below is what is said at the end of the fifth meeting, again before saying goodbye and meeting up six months later.

> You have made an important journey of reflection. We departed by the changes introduced into life by illness, by necessity to realize one's identity and find new important goals capable of giving meaning to life. We then examined, in the last meetings, how to concretely achieve one's goals effectively, finding the most useful ways to manage symptoms, emotions and communication. This is not only theoretical work of reflection, which in itself would be important, but included are provided materials and concrete approaches.
>
> What happens now? To use a metaphor, these two months were a bit of a sowing period. Now, it is a matter of applying oneself to germinate, and bear the fruit of all of this. For this to occur, it is best to do two things: The first is to continue to engage in the application of the themes and methods addressed: for this reason, participants have been provided with homework materials and directions to be followed. Include a vigorous insistence on the importance of the relaxation exercises: they are most helpful, and all of the participants sooner or later they learn to relax, as long as they do the exercises regularly. Then take back the material that was given to you and then do the same thing for the book, which really lends itself to being revisited for individual chapters, depending on your desire. The second thing to do is to try to put into practice what you know was indicated, but without anxiety. Everything must be done with great serenity and calm, without worry, but confident that today you have more tools than first to live better. Trust the reflection processes and adaptations that have been activated within you by having talked about important topics and examined concrete strategies. In the next meeting, we will return to these themes and methods examining together how these months have passed: the goals achieved, the difficulties encountered, the doubts, the new discoveries.

Sixth meeting

Box 3.11   Meeting 6 – follow-up: Review the experience

Introduction (1.)

- Fractional breathing, stabilization and centering of self

Contents and topics (2.)

- Review everything the process experienced, summarizing the contents that emerged
- Evaluation of changes carried out, habits modified and any difficulties encountered
- Focus: on which aspects each person wants to invest time and energy, to improve their quality of life further?

Conclusion (3.)

- Compilation of the questionnaire *Me and my life*
- Fractional breathing, stabilization and centering of self

The follow-up meeting: Review the experience

As customary, this meeting also opens with fractional breathing. Before moving on to practice, the facilitator reminds participants of the importance of establishing this type of exercise consistently to improve one's level of well-being.

After an initial moment where the participants tell how, in general, the six months in which they have not seen each other have passed, the group climate characterized by interaction between the members is reconstituted and the floor then passes to the facilitator to summarize the journey done together.

Thanks to the observation sheets compiled by the observer, who during the previous meetings had noted the contents that emerged meeting by meeting, and the key words summarized on the flipchart, it is possible for the facilitator to retrace the path taken together, underlining the salient aspects that emerged in each specific group. Therefore, even if the themes are the same for each group, it is possible to personalize the summary by enriching it with the examples and experiences that a particular group has expressed (see point 1 of Box 3.12). This helps the participants to retrace their experience from previous meetings, and each can bring to mind their past "psychological movements" and that of the group. The contribution of each participant is valued, as they feel recognized in the words reported by the facilitator.

Followed by introducing a few minutes of silence, the necessary time is left for the contents of the meeting to settle and everyone can reflect, in light of the path taken together, on what has changed or is changing since the time of their last meeting six months ago.

The participants are then invited to express their reflections aloud, which the facilitator writes down on the flip chart as each one contributes what they have to say. When the participants have finished, the facilitator once again reassumes what has been said, underlining the connections with the previous summary, so that the cognitive and emotional path of that group unfolds more and more clearly.

Once the content-related part has been concluded, the group is asked to fill out the *Me and my life* questionnaire (Appendix 4).

The meeting ends with relaxation exercises through breathing and we say good-bye and arrange an appointment in another six months.

Box 3.12   Sixth meeting: Points and tips for the facilitator

Below is the general summary that is proposed to the group and which is en-riched with the examples that each participant shared during the meetings.

> We are here to resume the dialogue and activities done together. It is an important journey that we have followed together, and we shall continue, bearing fruit over time.
>
> Briefly review what aspects were considered together in the group.
>
> In the first meeting, we had examined emotions and changes introduced by the disease, in many aspects of life. We learned breathing exercises, introducing fractional breathing.
>
> In the second meeting, we went on to observe who we are today, and what today may be able to give meaning to life (what can be important today, can make you feel achieved, can lead us to work hard to obtain it). In short, what reasons can we find to live as best we can, to ensure that existence is worth living in the main areas of our lives (emotional and family relationships, friendships, work, free time).
>
> In the third meeting, we examined how to achieve our own purposes, which are important to us and capable of giving meaning to life, effectively. To reach a concrete plan, we considered what they could be in the various contexts of our life the goals that are important to us, how we could achieve them, and how we could then evaluate whether all this had worked or if we needed to make some changes in the objectives or in ways. In particular, we looked at strategies and the tools that can be useful to achieve the objectives pre-established. We specifically evaluated the management of physical disorders, such as, in the case of fatigue, energy saving.
>
> In the fourth meeting, we considered effective methods to better manage emotions through positive circularity and we analyzed negative circularity; we also saw some rules for modulating emotions that are a source of suffering and to promote those related to

well-being. As for thoughts, we investigated the positive, negative and illusory ones, evaluating how each of them can bring us closer to or distance us from the perception of a good quality of life.

In the fifth meeting, we explored the benefits of good communication and the risks if the latter is not taken care sufficiently.

Let us take a look at:

- What has been most useful to you in recent months, among what had we seen together in the various meetings?
- Is there any particular aspect that you would like to review together today?
- What difficulties did you encounter in putting the instructions into practice?
- Were you able to engage in the proposed activities at home?

Let us then return to the requested themes... [space dedicated to these last]

Let us take a look at the steps to keep in mind when planning something.

- Ask yourself if the goals you are setting are important and meaningful to you, but at the same time attainable.
- Ask yourself what strategies, tools or aids can help you to achieve these objectives.
- Evaluate the result and make necessary adjustments.

Have there been any changes during this past period? If so, what kind?

In particular, it seems these are a few of the changes:

- the way you view yourself
- the objectives
- confidence in knowing how to deal with situations

Seventh meeting

The focus group meeting: Evaluation of the process

This meeting aims to evaluate the experience gained together with the participants, one year after the fifth meeting.

Attention is focused on how everyone experienced the process with respect to the organizational aspects and contents, for the personal perspective of the

Box 3.13   Meeting 7 – focus group: Evaluating the path

Introduction (1.)

- Breathing, stabilization and centering of self

Contents and topics (2.)

- Opinions on organizational aspects: timetable and place (convenience/inconvenience; extra-hospital context; adequacy of the room)
- Impressions on the topics treated: which ones are remembered, which ones are the most important and why, satisfaction with the level of in-depth study, opportunity for reflection for individual change; how they were experienced the exercises to do at home
- Analysis of the role played by group with respect to: discussion on the proposed themes, possibility of individual change
- Experience related to: questionnaire, material and homework, particularly in reference to eventual difficulties
- Replicability of the experience: Are there any adjustments to be made? If so, what would they be?
- Meeting with the neurologist for questions, doubts, in-depth study of topics

Conclusion (3.)

- Compilation of the questionnaire *Me and my life*
- Breathing, stabilization and centering of self

participants and any suggestions they may have, are essential to making changes and improvements in group activities to be proposed to newly diagnosed patients in the future (see point 1 of Box 3.14).

The thematic intersections explored during the meeting are the following.

1 Discussion on organizational aspects: when (time), place (convenience/ inconvenience; outside a hospital context; adequacy of the room).
2 Impressions regarding the topics covered: which ones are remembered, which ones are considered to have been most important and why, satisfaction with the level of in-depth analysis, opportunity for reflection for individual change; exercises to do at home (how were they experienced).
3 Analysis of the role played by the group with respect to: the discussion on the issues, the possibility of individual change.
4 Experiences relating to the questionnaire, the material and the homework, especially in reference to any difficulties encountered.
5 Replicability of the experience: if so, with what possible adjustments.

Once the information, suggestions and recommendations have been collected, the *Me and my life* questionnaire is administered for the fourth and final time.

The first part of the meeting ends with relaxation exercises through breathing.

The second part of the meeting is structured as a free space in which participants can ask all the questions they want to the neurologist responsible of the MS center.

This is a unique and precious opportunity in which a limited group of people have the opportunity to meet directly with the neurologist in charge of the center, including having adequate time available to ask questions and receive in-depth answers. This comparison allows a greater sense of control over one's illness and increases one's perception and one's feeling of self-efficacy.

Thanks to the people who make up the group and who have known each other for a year now, and the ability of the neurologist to put the participants at ease through a warm and welcoming human approach, an extremely pleasant and productive relational climate is created.

The questions generally focus on research developments on MS and any therapeutic innovations. The discussion continues with more personal questions regarding the management of therapies and requests for clarification on specific areas ranging from bureaucratic aspects to requests for insights on symptomatic therapies and complementary therapies, such as nutrition and physical activity.

The neurologist also takes advantage of the opportunity to ask the point of view of each of the participants on their experience they have had with the MS center. In this way, the neurologist collects important feedback from those who make access the specialist neurological clinic, this is very helpful for understanding if and how it is possible to improve the services offered. Furthermore, it has the possibility to explain why some procedures have to be done in a certain way (particularly bureaucratic protocols), since it is not uncommon for someone to complain about the time used to adapt to the required procedures.

Finally, part of the time is dedicated to presenting and explaining the research in progress, both in general all that is being carried out by various research groups on MS and, specifically, that conducted by the CReSM research group.

The conclusion of the meeting is often a time particularly full of enthusiasm, an exchange of experiences and points of view in where it is possible to notice the changes that have occurred on an individual level; a clearer constructive attitude, each showing a far less sense of desolation and destructivity toward their illness.

Since many participants in the groups have expressed the desire to continue meeting after the conclusion of the intervention project, informal meetings have been organized over the years, always at the Miradolo Castle headquarters, both on the occasion of Christmas greetings and to meet the managers of the Cosso Foundation and learn about its history and activities. At the same time, other people organized themselves independently to meet in other moments of leisure after the end of the program.

Box 3.14   Seventh meeting: Points and tips for the facilitator

Below are the traces of the meeting.

Welcome to this meeting. As we have expressed to you, this meeting aims to evaluate together the path taken: given we have shared an important and new experience together, we wish to understand together with you, if it is fine as it is from an organizational perspective including information provided, and most importantly, is it helpful for you and are there specifics that need to be changed or modified? This way we will be able to improve activities in the future. Your insight and your suggestions are indispensable, because you have and give firsthand experience, from the inside, and therefore no one else if not you, are able to evaluate it.

Let's start with the organizational aspects, seeing what from your perspective was effective and what does not:

- hours;
- frequency of meetings and their number and
- place (convenience/inconvenience; non-hospital context; adequacy cleanliness of the room).

Let's now move on to your impressions on the topics covered:

- which ones do you remember most;
- which ones in your opinion were most important and useful in general;
- more specifically, what were useful opportunities for reflection for your individual change;

- which ones have been useful for your daily life;
- which ones did you struggle the most in dealing with? which ones were fatiguing for you?
- were there topics covered that made you feel anxious or generated tension, anger or desire in you to stop coming to the group? What were they? and
- how satisfied are you with the level of in-depth analysis.

Let us now consider the material gradually provided. Do you remember which materials were given to you?

Let's evaluate those:

- clarity, understandability and
- usefulness and real use.

Let's also look at exercises to do at home. Do you remember which exercises you have been asked to do?

Evaluate:

- how they were experienced (as useful, as an imposition, etc.) and
- if they were done or not.

Let us now address an important aspect, which concerns the group, that is, the role played by the group as such, to be together with other people who are different but share the same illness.

Let's see together how you experienced it, in particular with respect to:

- the discussion on the proposed topics (if therefore being in a group has facilitated the in-depth analysis, if the comparison with others has helped you understand yourself, or if you felt confusion, was it distracting to worry about what someone else says);
- emotions (fear of talking about oneself or expressing one's opinion, irritation toward someone in the group, poor harmony, climate positive);
- the possibility of individual change (if therefore the group has stimulated change in you and why, for example, given the comparison) and
- specifically, did you have the desire to leave the group? What prompted you to continue?

During the meetings, questionnaires were submitted to you. Let's see how this experience was for you and in particular whether it posed any difficulties for you, and which ones.

Thinking of proposing this activity to other people who have recently been diagnosed with MS, are there adjustments or changes you are interested in proposing?

References

Bonino, S. (2021). *Coping with chronic illness. Theories, issues and lived experiences.* Routledge.

Briones-Buixassa, L., Milà, R. M., Aragonès, J., Bufill, E., Olaya, B., & Arrufat, F. X. (2015). Stress and multiple sclerosis: A systematic review considering potential moderating and mediating factors and methods of assessing stress. *Health Psychology Open*, *2*(2), Article 2055102915612271.

Grice, P. (1989). *Studies in the way of words.* Harvard University Press.

Solari, A., Acquarone, N., Pucci, E., Martinelli, V., Marrosu, M. G., Trojano, M., Borreani, C., & Messmer Uccelli, M. (2007). Communicating the diagnosis of multiple sclerosis - a qualitative study. *Multiple Sclerosis*, *13*, 763–769.

Thompson, C. M., Pulido, M. D., Babu, S., Zenzola, N., & Chiu, C. (2022). Communication between persons with multiple sclerosis and their health care providers: A scoping review. *Patient Education and Counseling*, *105*(12), 3341–3368.

4 Between theory and intervention

The contribution of the research

Federica Graziano and Emanuela Calandri

Introduction

One of the main features of this project is the centrality of research as inquiry both for increasing knowledge of the disease in its psychological aspects and for the evaluation of the interventions proposed. Research represents the tool for holding together theory and intervention, as a kind of "red thread", in a circular process that moves from theory to intervention and from intervention back to theory. As already pointed out in Chapter 1, this constitutes an important strength of the project.

The intervention is grounded in solid theoretical foundations, a necessary starting point, especially given the novelty of the issues addressed. Theory is constantly confronted with people's lived experience throughout the course of the intervention project. The data collected during the intervention, through questionnaires, focus groups and interviews, served both for the evaluation of the effectiveness of the intervention itself and for the theoretical investigation of the psychological constructs that represent its foundation. The data derived from the evaluation and theoretical deepening have in turn suggested modifications and additions to the activities proposed and opened new avenues of intervention.

This chapter will outline the stages of this project, which runs in a circular way between theory and intervention. In the first stage, a pilot project was conducted and evaluated through comparison between an intervention group and a comparison group; the results confirmed the effectiveness of the intervention with respect to different areas of patients' life experience (see the section *The pilot project*). In addition, the data collected through the pilot project allowed us to have confirmation of the validity of the theoretical model underlying the intervention, particularly about the links between identity, self-efficacy and sense of coherence and the role that these factors have on adjustment to illness (see the paragraph *The role of identity, sense of coherence and self-efficacy for the adjustment to the illness*).

The data collected in this first phase finally enabled the validation of a new and agile instrument to assess self-efficacy in the management of multiple sclerosis (MS) (see the section *Self-efficacy in the management of MS: A novel assessment tool*).

From the set of these results, a second phase of the project specifically focused on newly diagnosed patients (people who had been diagnosed with MS within the

DOI: 10.4324/9781003484400-4

last three years) was planned and implemented. This project was also evaluated for effectiveness through comparison between an intervention group and a comparison group, and the results confirmed the validity of the project, with results overlapping with those obtained in the first phase (see the paragraph *The project for newly diagnosed patients*). In addition, the data collected on newly diagnosed patients made it possible to conduct theoretical insight into some aspects of living with chronic illness that have been little investigated in the literature. In particular, the role of coping strategies for adjustment to the illness in the first years after diagnosis (see *The role of coping strategies and sense of coherence for the adjustment to illness in newly diagnosed patients*), the experience of illness in young adults and the role of identity (see the paragraph *Identity and MS: The double challenge of the newly diagnosed young adult*) and the experience of the illness in women and the role of motherhood (see the section *MS in women: Identity and the role of motherhood in newly diagnosed women*).

These insights made it possible to refine the content proposed in the group meetings, as well as to design new lines of intervention focused, on the one hand, on the parents of young adult patients and, on the other, on parents with MS. The main results of the research work conducted at the various stages will be presented below, indicating the scientific articles in which they were published, whose abstracts are given in Appendix 6.

The pilot project

As outlined in Chapter 1, the evaluation of a psychological intervention is a complex but necessary process to understand whether it is going in the right direction and what changes, if any, need to be made. The evaluation involves dealing not only with the complexity of the constructs to be evaluated, but also with people's concrete life experiences, including the many variables that come into play in each person's daily living. In the specific case of our project, when we conducted this first evaluation (in the years between 2010 and 2012), a few benchmark studies were available in the literature, because it was a completely new approach in terms of characteristics and objectives. To conduct an integrated evaluation that took this complexity into account, we used different tools. For the evaluation of the effectiveness of the intervention, we compared patients who had participated in the groups (i.e., intervention group, consisting of 41 people) and those who had not participated (i.e., comparison group, composed of 41 people). The patients who had followed the groups ranged in age from 26 to 64 years (with a mean of 42 years, standard deviation 8.5 years) and were divided into six groups according to age group (20–35 years, 36–50 years, 50+ years). Sixty-six percent were women and disease duration ranged from 1 to 22 years (mean duration 8.6 years, standard deviation 5.2 years). As described above, the pilot project consisted of four meetings. The patients in the comparison attended three information meetings on MS that covered, respectively: new treatments, alternative and complementary therapies and nutrition. The activity was held in plenary. The age of the patients in the comparison group ranged from 21 to 57 years (with a mean of 38 years, standard deviation 10 years), 60% were women, and the duration of disease ranged from 1 to 22 years (mean duration 7.2 years, standard deviation 5.3 years; for details of the study, see Graziano et al., 2014).

The evaluation of effectiveness was based on data obtained from the questionnaire *Me and my life* completed by participants at four points in time (before the intervention, at the completion of the four meetings, at six months and at one year). Through these questionnaires, change over time was assessed through a series of variables on which we hypothesized that the intervention would have an impact (see Box 4.1). In addition, the evaluation took into account information obtained

---

Box 4.1   Psychological constructs investigated in the questionnaire *Me and my life*: Measures and description

The variables investigated through the *Me and my life* questionnaire are presented below along with the measures used for their evaluation. Some variables refer to the psychological aspects on which the intervention is focused (identity, sense of coherence, self-efficacy in managing MS) or to other relevant aspects in the way of coping with the illness (coping strategies), while other variables represent indicators of the expected outcomes of the intervention (quality of life, depressive symptoms, psychological well-being and optimism). The complete questionnaire is provided in Appendix 4.

Identity

The identity construct has been investigated with reference to the Motivated Identity Construction Theory (Vignoles, 2011; Vignoles et al., 2006). According to this model, the definition of identity is guided by the following six psychological motives, defined as "identity motives":

- self-esteem: the motivation of individuals to represent themselves in a positive way;
- efficacy: the motivation to feel competent and capable of influencing one's environment;
- continuity: the motivation to preserve a sense of continuity over time, despite the changes experienced throughout life;
- belongingness: the motivation to maintain a sense of closeness to other people within one's social context;
- distinctiveness: the need to differentiate oneself from others and assert one's uniqueness and
- meaning: the need to perceive that life is endowed with significance.

Greater satisfaction in the above-listed "identity motives" leads to greater satisfaction with one's identity. Identity was then assessed through the Identity Motives Scale (Manzi et al., 2010), which investigates the six identity motives through twelve questions (two for each motive) worded in a positive sense (e.g., "When I think about my future I think I will feel proud": satisfaction with self-esteem) or negative (e.g., "When I think about my future I think I will feel powerless": threat to self-esteem), rated on a scale from 1 (extremely disagree) to 5 (extremely agree). When we evaluate "identity satisfaction," we refer to the total score of the six subscales (i.e., the six identity motives, with the negative items recoded in reverse) obtained by summing the answers given to all questions by each person. The range of scores is between 12 and 60; higher scores correspond to greater identity satisfaction.

Sense of coherence

Sense of coherence was assessed through the Sense of Coherence (SOC) scale (Antonovsky, 1993); it consists of 11 items assessed on a 7-point scale with anchoring categories specific for each item (e.g., the question "For you, doing everyday things is an occasion for..." involves a response on the 7-point scale ranging from "suffering and boredom" to "pleasure and satis-faction"; the question "How often do you feel that there is little meaning in the things you do in everyday life?" involves a response on the 7-point scale ranging from "never" to "very often"). The range of scores is from 11 to 77; higher scores represent the perception of a greater sense of coherence.

Self-efficacy in dealing with MS

See Box 4.6

Coping strategies

Coping strategies were assessed through three subscales of the Coping with Multiple Sclerosis Scale (CMSS) (Pakenham, 2001):

- Problem solving (five items, e.g., "I thought about how I could have best solve the problem"), range 5–25;
- Emotional coping (three items, e.g., "I was able to express my emotions"), range 3–15 and
- Avoidance (four items, e.g., "I made sure not to think about it"), range 4–20.

People should indicate how many times in the past month they have used each strategy to cope with the difficulties of MS, on a scale of 1 (never) to 5 (very often).

Quality of life

Quality of life was assessed through the SF-12 Health Survey (Ware et al., 1995), consisting of 12 items that provide two measures, one referred to as physical health (e.g., "Does your health currently limit you to climbing a few floors of stairs?" which can be answered "Yes, a lot", "Yes, partially", "No, not at all") and the other as mental health (e.g., "In the last four weeks, how long have you felt calm and peaceful?" which can be answered on a scale from 1, which indicates "always", to 6, which indicates "never"). The standardized score for each scale has a range between 0 and 100. When we talk about "quality of life", we refer to the sum of the scores obtained in the two subscales of physical health and mental health.

Depressive symptoms

Depressive symptoms were assessed through the Center for Epidemiologic Studies Depression Scale (CES-D) in the 10-item short form (Andresen et al., 1994): it assesses the frequency of depressive symptoms in the previous week on a scale from 0 (rarely or never) to 3 (always or almost always) (example item, "I have been worried about some things that I am generally not worried about"). The range of scores is between 0 and 30. The cutoff for talking about a significant presence of depressive symptoms is 10.

Affective well-being

Affective well-being was assessed through the Positive and Negative Affect Schedule (PANAS) (Terracciano et al., 2003; Watson et al., 1988). It comprises two mood scales: positive affect (PA) (10 items, e.g., interested, enthusiastic) and negative affect (NA) (10 items, e.g., scared, nervous); each item is rated on a 5-point scale (from 1 "never" to 5 "always") to indicate the number of times the respondent feels in the way described by each adjective in their daily living. The range of scores is from −40 e +50.

When we address:

- "positive affect" refers to the sum of the positive adjectives;
- "negative affect" refers to the sum of the negative adjectives and
- "affective well-being" refers to the score derived from positive affect minus negative affect.

Optimism

Optimism was evaluated through the LOT-R (Chiesi et al., 2013; Scheier et al., 1994), a scale assessing the disposition to optimism through 10 items, three positive (e.g., "In difficult times I expect everything to work out for the best"), three negative (e.g., "I almost never expect things to turn out for the best") and four fillers (i.e., questions that do not contribute to the final score, e.g., "I derive a lot of satisfaction from being with my friends"). The Likert response scale ranges from 1 (strongly disagree) to 5 (strongly agree). The range of the scores is between 6 and 30; higher scores indicate greater optimism.

from the participants' satisfaction questionnaire for the intervention in which they had participated (*My point of view* questionnaire; see Box 4.2), from the observation of the meetings (see Box 4.3), from the audio-recording and subsequent content analysis of the meetings, and from the concluding focus group, one year after the completion of the four meetings (see Figure 4.1, Timing and measurement tools).

An initial indication of the project's success comes from the data on participation over time. Group psychological support interventions require great commitment from participants, not only in terms of their willingness to "get involved" and engage with others, but also because of the need to reconcile participation in the group with daily life commitments, already made more difficult by one's illness. For this reason, often interventions of this type are characterized by a high dropout rate over time, as the meetings continue. In contrast, in our intervention the dropout rate is low; in fact, only 12% of participants dropped out before the end of the four meetings and 34% did not participate in the six-month follow-up. Our intervention was thus characterized by significant retention over time. The data drawn from the satisfaction questionnaire (*My point of view*) completed at the end of the four meetings returned a very positive overall assessment of the course: in particular, 80% of the participants expressed a positive or very positive response regarding their experience, 63% found it to be a useful or very useful experience, all would repeat the experience or recommend it to other patients, and 64% reported a positive change in their feelings and attitudes. In the space for comments, where we ask patients

---

Box 4.2 The participants' satisfaction questionnaire (*My point of view*)

At the end of the four group sessions (see "POST-TEST – T2" in Figure 4.1), participants complete the *My point of view* questionnaire, which contains a series of questions about their satisfaction with the sessions, their usefulness, positive aspects and critical issues. Space is left in the questionnaire to indicate any difficulties and useful suggestions for the working group to improve the intervention. The questionnaire is given in its entirety in Appendix 5.

Box 4.3   The observation of the sessions

In each of the group sessions, the facilitator is joined by an observer. The observer is guided by an observation grid on which he/she takes note of both the content expressed by the participants and a range of nonverbal information (the disposition of the participants, the emotional tone of the interventions made by each of them, their body posture, the direction of their gazes). The grid includes a section of concluding observations, with an assessment of the group climate, participants' attitudes and their experiences with the group. The information gleaned from the observation is crucial for the facilitator to return later to analyze the session and appropriately modulate the conduct of the program in the following session and in the follow-up. They are also important for the working group, as a tool for process evaluation and for planning possible modifications and additions to the program of intervention.

The observation grid is given in full in Appendix 3.

to report critical issues or suggestions, several participants reported the usefulness of implementing this type of intervention in the early years of illness, when one needs insight and understanding on how to cope with their overwhelming sense of bewilderment as a consequence of one's diagnosis.

The results of the statistical analysis of the data collected with the questionnaire *Me and my life* made it possible to highlight how the intervention had a significant impact on quality of life, which at six-month follow-up was higher in the people who had participated in the group meetings compared to those who had attended

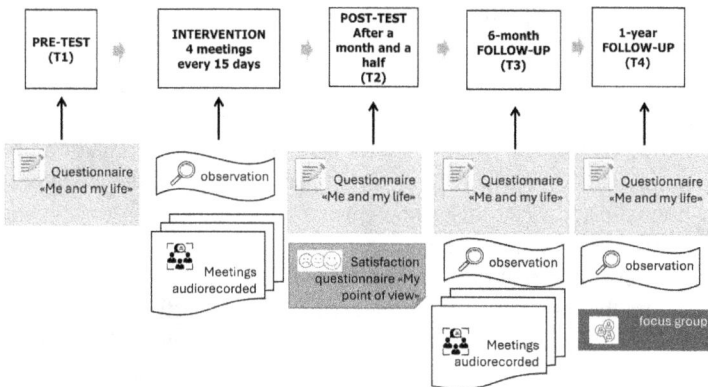

Figure 4.1 Pilot project: Timing and measurement tools.

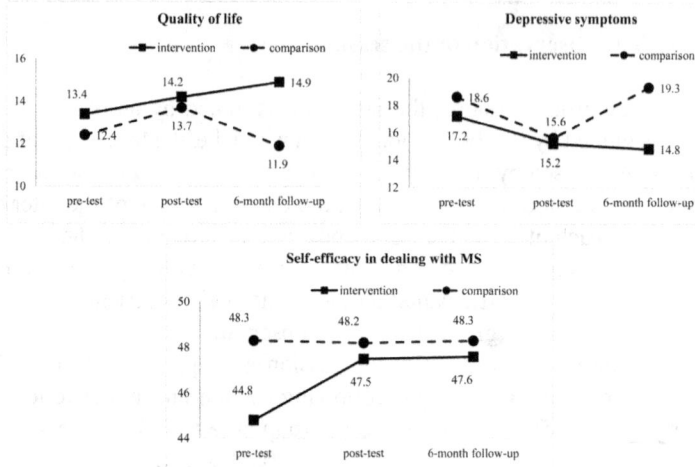

Figure 4.2 Evaluation of effectiveness of the pilot intervention (mean scores of quality of life, depressive symptoms and self-efficacy in dealing with MS in the intervention group and comparison group).

Note: Quality of life was assessed by a 9-item scale taken from MSQOL-54 (Multiple Sclerosis Quality of Life; Solari et al., 1999) and the range of the scale is 0 to 24. Depressive symptoms were assessed through the CES-D-20 (Center for Epidemiologic Studies Depression 20-item scale; Fava, 1983) and the range of the scale is 0 to 60. The cutoff for the presence of significant depressive symptoms is 16.

the informational meetings. Six months after the intervention, patients who had attended the groups tended to report fewer depressive symptoms and greater psychological well-being. Furthermore, at the conclusion of the four-meeting course, people who had attended the groups reported greater perceived self-efficacy in disease management compared with baseline scores, and they maintained favorable levels of self-efficacy over time (see Figure 4.2).

The follow-up focus group conducted one year after the conclusion of the intervention series investigated the participants' views on the experience of the group course, the usefulness of the topics covered, the way the meetings were conducted, and the materials provided. The participants' words allowed us to "flesh out" the data that emerged from the questionnaires and confirm a positive assessment of the experience, as well as offering useful insights for the continuation of this intervention approach. In particular, all participants recognized the usefulness of the group to compare and share their experience; moreover, it emerged how the group fostered motivation to pursue experiences of change.

Many participants noted that the time available to cover the various topics was too limited and that more meetings are needed. Several participants suggested that this course be systematized, to be implemented when people receive a diagnosis of MS. Finally, the need emerged to include a meeting with a neurologist in this pathway exploring issues and concerns that are often not addressed in individual outpatient visits (see Box 4.5).

Box 4.4   The participants' words. Some considerations from the focus groups of the pilot project

The following are some examples of considerations that emerged by patients during the focus groups held at the end of the sessions of the pilot project. For the participants, the group meetings were an opportunity for discussion, sharing and mutual support.

> *It was interesting to see how others dealt with the same problem (woman, youth group 20-35 years old).*
> *You feel relaxed here because you can talk freely. It is a mutual exchange (woman, adult group 36-50 years old).*
> *With some people who have the same problem there is a different dialogue: authentic and constructive (man, adult group over 50 years old).*

Some admit that it was an exhausting experience, others wish they had more time on their hands.

> *Sometimes I come out mentally exhausted because you go digging for past stories. After the first meeting I left here and wondered whether to come back or not (man, adult group 36-50 years old).*
> *Besides enjoying the company, I would have enjoyed a few more meetings... maybe they would have been good and even a little bad, but it is an important thing (woman, youth group 20-35 years old)*

Some participants report experiences of change following participation in the groups.

> *In my opinion it was good because I disclosed the disease to [...]; for me it is already so much because I never told anyone (man, adult group 36-50 years old).*
> *When it came to talking about having a goal, moving forward, I realized that I had forgotten what a goal was. I was living a bit by the day. Now, a year later, I feel much more determined (woman, adult group over 50).*
> *Now even if you have bad times, you have more resources to deal with them (woman, youth group 20-35 years old).*
> *It is always problematic for me to be able to take the injection because I am a little afraid, then comparing how to do it with other people made me feel better (woman, adult group 36-50 years old).*

Several aspects addressed in the groups were appreciated and found useful.

> *The fact of not wasting energy on unattainable goals. Avoiding dwelling on things you can no longer change (woman, adult group 36-50 years old).*

> *For example, breathing exercises have been a very positive thing. Always starting with those helped me a lot and currently I still use them. It is something valuable, a practical tool that I use a lot (woman, youth group 20-35 years old).*
>
> *For example, the contribution "Small rules to manage emotions that are a source of suffering and encourage positive ones." It is very concise, very practical. These things are beautiful because you flip through them and read half a page and it gives you something. That's exactly what it takes (woman, adult group over 50).*

Box 4.5   The process of change in the words of the participants

The following are some phrases that emerged during the sessions that represent examples of mechanisms of resistance to change and openness to change (for a detailed discussion, see Borghi et al., 2018).

Resistance to change

During the meeting regarding the theme of identity, when asked by the facilitator about what gave meaning to one's life before the diagnosis and about what gives meaning today, one participant expresses his resistance with an aggressive tone and demonstrating denial:

> *It is very difficult to interpret the question [...] the disease has not changed anything, what made sense to me before makes sense even today... by the way I do not call it a disease but a health problem [...] I cannot connect the disease to this discourse [of meaning] (man, youth group 20-35 years old).*

During the session on self-efficacy, when asked by the facilitator about how to be able to redefine goals in a particular area and find appropriate strategies to achieve them, one participant avoided the question stating:

> *It is better not to make plans! (man, youth group 20-35 years old).*

During the sessions, the discussion sometimes brings out negative emotions and some participants shift the discussion to topics that are not strictly relevant but may be more reassuring. For example, while a participant is talking about how to handle therapy when one has to travel, a woman suddenly says:

> *But how do you do interferon? Do you do it when you are sick? I have never done it! (woman, adult group 36-50 years old).*

Openness to change

Participants' words reveal an intention to enact a change in line with the goals of the intervention; some of them tell of a change that has already occurred as a result of the group experience:

> *My goal is to be able to feel good ... doing what I can, for example, if I am tired, I would like to be able to say it, without feeling guilty about it (woman, adult group, over 50).*
>
> *I have to work on the rules of good communication, I don't always tell it like it is, maybe sometimes it bothers me to admit [...] I feel like everyone has to notice. I have to be a little clearer... (woman, youth group 20-35 years old).*
>
> *To me [breathing] helps a lot, it calms me down: it is one of the aspects I have appreciated most in these meetings (man, adult group over 50).*
>
> *For me personally, it helped to come here to be less impulsive than I am, in the sense that, I have changed, I am a little more thoughtful, I used to act immediately, instead now I reason more before acting (woman, adult group 36-50 years old).*
>
> *These meetings allowed me to see things in a more positive way...I thought about how important it is to reorganize time, without using rigid patterns (woman, adult group over 50).*
>
> *I, for example, never told anyone [about the disease], that is, very few people know about it and recently instead I told to [...] Yes, I liked it, I didn't expect something like that. It was better than what I expected (woman, adult group 36-50 years old).*

The evaluation of both effectiveness and satisfaction has therefore demonstrated that the group intervention was useful because it contributed to the comparison and sharing of experiences among people, it fostered mutual support, had a significant effect in increasing the perceived self-efficacy in managing the disease and overall contributed to improving quality of life and adjustment.

The evaluation of the pilot project, in addition to analyzing data obtained from the questionnaires and focus groups, it was also based on audio-recordings and related transcripts of the content that emerged during the patient group meetings. The

analysis of the content that emerged in the groups was an onerous and a very challenging task, but also a fundamental tool for examining in-depth patients' thinking
about the course taken and to understand their process of change over the course
of the meetings. These results completed the evaluation process by providing a
detailed and complex picture (for details, see Borghi et al., 2018). Analysis of the
meetings content revealed the theme of change as central, clearly expressed by
participants in its dual valence of resistance to change, on the one hand, and openness to change, on the other.

In particular, resistance to change was most present at the beginning of the
course, i.e., during the first and second group meetings; this result was expected,
since the participants were facing a new experience (i.e., that of a group intervention) toward which they may have had positive expectations, but also fears.
However, over the course of the meetings, the patients reported a gradual and
significant openness to change that was unfolding over time. Indeed, openness to
change became increasingly evident with a "peak" in the middle of the course,
when a comfortable climate had been created in the group, considering particularly
relevant topics had already been addressed and discussed. Interestingly, during all
of the meetings, participants' resistance never completely disappeared: indeed, this
is a challenging and often difficult path, in the presence of a chronic disease with
significant consequences. The fact that openness to change remained constant at
the six-month follow-up, although with a slight decline during the last intervention meeting, this suggests that participants changed aspects of themselves and
maintained these changes even after the intervention ended (see Figure 4.3 and

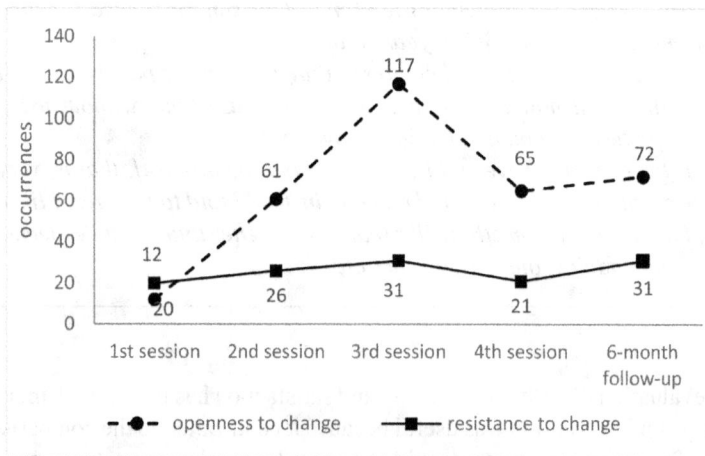

Figure 4.3 Openness to change and resistance to change during the group sessions of the
pilot project.

Note: Results of the content analysis carried out on the text obtained from the transcripts of the audio-
recordings. On the vertical axis are the occurrences, that is, the number of sentences referring, respectively, to openness to change and resistances, which emerged in each meeting.

Box 4.5). These results not only confirmed those obtained from the questionnaires, but actually expanded them. In fact, through the words of the participants we captured the impact of the intervention on different aspects of their quality of life, more detailed and nuanced than their responses to the questionnaire provided. Participants' words also enabled us to capture the effect of the intervention on such areas as redefining identity and meaning of life after diagnosis. These are in fact complex and subtle aspects that a questionnaire often fails to capture, when on the contrary come to light when conducting an in-depth analysis of the contents that emerged during the meetings.

From a more general point of view, all of the aspects outlined above highlight the importance of assessing the effectiveness of a psychological intervention through various tools to capture different aspects: questionnaires, with closed questions and validated measures that allow for robustness from a statistical point of view and the possibility of comparison with the results of other studies published in the literature; focus groups, which allow interaction among participants capable of revealing new elements from the comparison and the analysis of the content of verbalizations, which allows to grasp the specificity of the individual experiences.

From a specific point of view, the objectives of our project in the preliminary phase confirmed the validity of our proposal both methodologically and in terms of content. From the words of the participants and from the analysis of the meetings, confirms the usefulness of the intervention group in fostering discussion and change. Analysis of the questionnaires and meetings revealed the effectiveness of intervention in reducing depressive symptoms hence promoting a better quality of life, prompting the ability to cope with one's chronic illness and higher psychological well-being. At the same time, this validation phase suggested a number of modifications regarding the continuation of our activities: first, the decision to design an intervention specifically aimed at newly diagnosed individuals (see the paragraph devoted to that project, later in the chapter). As already explained in Chapter 1, this choice was motivated by both the analysis of the literature and by our clinical experience and was further confirmed by the data that emerged in the pilot project. The first three years after diagnosis represent a critical period that is often underestimated. This is why an intervention approach targeting all newly diagnosed patients is needed, to empower them to cope as one can from the time of diagnosis, acquiring functional ways to deal with the challenges of chronic illness and establishing an awareness of the need for continuous adaptation over the years. The changes to the project did not affect the topics of the meetings nor the methodology, but only the outline for conducting them, considering the specificity of the illness experience for a person a few years after diagnosis. In addition, we chose to divide the intervention into five meetings. As emerged from our experience, as well as from the evaluation of the participants and the analysis of the content of the meetings, there was often insufficient time to fully address all topics, especially those related to the management of emotions and communication. In addition, there had sometimes been a feeling that the group experience had been interrupted too early and that there was a need to have more time to conclude the course. Moreover, from our point of view having one more meeting available would have allowed us to structure the group better at the beginning of the course in order to take full advantage of its potential. Finally, again based on the participants' observations, we decided to devote the final meeting one year after the intervention process partly to the focus group and partly to meeting with a neurologist, to whom participants can address any questions of a more strictly medical nature, and in particular questions about symptoms, medication management, and new therapies. The possibility of having this information represents for patients an aid in facing the disease also from a psychological point of view, increasing their perception of self-efficacy and control over the disease (Bonino, 2021). Intervention by the neurologist is closely related to issues addressed during meetings and represents a completion of the group course, in a conceptional way in which body and psyche, knowledge and emotions and medical and psychological intervention are inextricably linked.

The role of identity, sense of coherence and self-efficacy for the adjustment to illness

As mentioned in the introduction, the data we collected through questionnaires during the pilot project served not only to assess the effectiveness of the intervention, but also to theoretically explore in greater depth the psychological constructs underlying it. In particular, the data collected before the start of the course, both in the intervention group and in the comparison group ("PRE-TEST – T2" in Figure 4.1), allowed us to have descriptive information about the sample of patients involved and to investigate the links between the variables assessed (for details, see Calandri et al., 2019). In terms of descriptive data, 65% of patients have symptoms of depression, which is in line with other works in the literature highlighting that depression is a widespread issue among people with MS (Peres et al., 2022). Psychological well-being and quality of life are lower than the levels observed in the healthy population (Klevan et al., 2014; McCabe & McKern, 2002). Specifically, our data indicate the presence of higher depressive symptoms among young adults (aged 20–35 years) and among those who have been diagnosed for less than three years than those with a longer history of the disease.

In addition, depressive symptoms are higher among those who are not working than among those who are gainfully employed. These data deserve some reflections. First, the period following diagnosis, which often affects people in young adulthood, is confirmed as particularly difficult, in terms of negative emotional experiences. As highlighted, these difficulties are especially evident among patients who are not working, regardless of age: they are likely to experience greater difficulties either because they often live with a condition of illness that does not allow them to work, or because they are missing a dimension of life that plays an important role in defining one's identity and constructing meaning. We observed that those with family burdens, particularly those with children, report experiencing lower levels of psychological well-being than those who live alone. The presence of a family, while it can be a source of emotional support, also poses a more difficult burden and commitment to cope with one's disease, especially considering that many patients are women with minor children; this topic will be explored

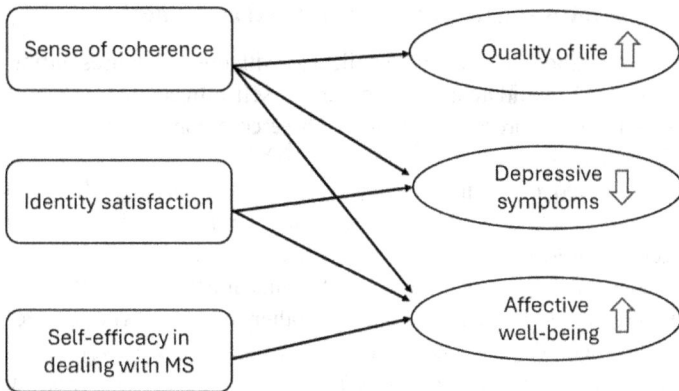

Figure 4.4 Relationships between personal variables (sense of coherence, identity satisfaction and self-efficacy in dealing with MS) and adjustment to the illness (quality of life, depressive symptoms and affective well-being).

specifically in the paragraph *MS in women: Identity and the role of motherhood in newly diagnosed women.*

Depression and well-being are also related to the personal variables considered; in fact, good levels of identity satisfaction, sense of coherence and self-efficacy in dealing with illness are accompanied by greater well-being, higher quality of life and fewer depressive symptoms. We report below in more detail the relationships that emerged among the variables considered (Figure 4.4).

- The sense of coherence is related to fewer depressive symptoms, greater psychological well-being and higher quality of life, particularly regarding the psychological component (mental health).
- Identity satisfaction is related to fewer depressive symptoms and higher psychological well-being.
- Self-efficacy in managing MS is related to greater psychological well-being.

Taken together, these results highlight the relevance of the three separate variables for the adjustment to illness. The sense of coherence seems to be the dimension that binds across all domains, confirming how the ability to find meaning in one's life experience is important for adaptation to illness. The redefinition of one's identity is confirmed as a central aspect, particularly with respect to emotional experiences, protecting against depressive feelings and promoting psychological well-being. Finally, self-efficacy in dealing with one's illness – thus feeling capable to set meaningful and achievable goals and manage symptoms – is related to the positive dimension of adaptation, represented by psychological well-being. The specificity of self-efficacy will be discussed in greater detail in the next paragraph.

Self-efficacy in the management of MS: A novel assessment tool

As stated in the introduction, the data collected with questionnaires during the pilot project were used to validate a new measure of self-efficacy in one's management of MS. Self-efficacy represents one of the three core constructs of our theoretical model of intervention.

When we started designing the intervention and thinking about assessment tools, we found several examples of scales in the literature to assess self-efficacy in the management of MS; however, each one had limitations.

Some scales assessed effectiveness in the management of chronic diseases in general or were related to chronic diseases other than MS, whereas we were interested in the specificity of this disease. Other measures were related to MS, but narrowly focused on self-efficacy in exercising physical activity (Schwartz et al., 1996), whereas we were interested in a broader measure that included different aspects of daily management of the disease. Other scales also took psychological aspects into account, but they were presented as scales of attitude rather than perception of ability (Airlie et al., 2001; Rigby et al., 2003). From these considerations, we decided to formulate a new measure that would have the following characteristics:

1   To be specific to patients with MS, given the peculiarity of the symptoms and characteristics of this disease compared with other chronic conditions.
2   To take into account both physical and psychological aspects related to the disease.
3   To measure perceived ability in specific areas and not generic attitudes.

In addition, we wanted to develop a scale that was short, easy to administer by psychologists, neurologists or other professionals, and especially agile to be filled out by patients, taking into account the fatigue they already experience due to their illness, which may be exacerbated by the presentation of long batteries of questions. A tool with these characteristics can be useful not only for research purposes, but also for clinical application, where one intends to assess the psychological resources of the individual patient, or if one wants to evaluate the effectiveness of an intervention aimed at enhancing self-efficacy. To construct this scale, we relied on both existing scales and the information that came to us directly from patients and from the experience of other professionals who work closely with them. This work led to the formulation of a battery of 15 questions assessing perceived self-efficacy in two areas, namely, in goal setting and in symptom management (see Box 4.6). These are two crucial aspects that constitute the sense of efficacy of patients: on the one hand, the ability to set goals and plan the daily activities in relation to the limitations and possibilities of the disease, on the other hand, the ability to manage physical symptoms and related psychological difficulties. They are expected to have positive effects on the adjustment and psychological well-being of patients.

Statistical analyses for the validation of this scale were conducted on a sample of 203 patients (mean age 40 years, 66% female, 95% with a relapsing–remitting

Box 4.6   The scale of self-efficacy in dealing with MS (SEMS, Self-Efficacy in MS scale; Bonino et al., 2018)

The following statements describe some situations that can be difficult to control. Please indicate how much you feel confident to deal with each situation, by putting an X on the number which best expresses your feeling (1 = ot at all confident; 2 = a little confident; 3 = quite confident; 4 = very confident; 5 = extremely confident).

1. Take control over negative feelings (e.g., sadness, anger, anxiety)	1	2	3	4	5
2. Organize the day and week time to reduce fatigue	1	2	3	4	5
3. Find the way to do what it is important for me in the family	1	2	3	4	5
4. Find the way to do what it is important for me in my job and social life	1	2	3	4	5
5. Find the way to do what it is important for me with my friends	1	2	3	4	5
6. Find the way to do what it is important for me during free time	1	2	3	4	5
7. Setting new goals	1	2	3	4	5
8. Find the way to reach goals	1	2	3	4	5
9. Overcome the obstacles due to physical difficulties and disabilities	1	2	3	4	5
10. Find the way to reduce the appearance and seriousness of physical disturbances	1	2	3	4	5
11. Recognize what I can do in spite of physical limitations	1	2	3	4	5
12. Not get discouraged because of unexpected events	1	2	3	4	5
13. Search for support and help from others when I need it	1	2	3	4	5
14. Voice my desires and preferences to family, friends, and colleagues	1	2	3	4	5
15. Deal with day-to-day life in an autonomous way despite difficulties	1	2	3	4	5

Items 2, 3, 4, 5, 6, 7, 8, 13 and 14 constitute the goal setting factor, while items 1, 9, 10, 11, 12 and 15 constitute the symptoms management factor. The range of the scale is between 15 and 75. This material can be found in the questionnaire *Me and my life* (Appendix 4).

form of MS, with an EDSS between 1 and 5.5, indicating mild-to-moderate disability, and an average duration of disease of about six years) and showed that this scale structure, with the two factors "goal setting" (nine items) and "symptom management" (six items) has satisfactory psychometric properties (for details, see Bonino et al., 2018). Statistical analyses conducted to assess the validity of the measure showed that higher self-efficacy scores on both factors are related to a greater sense of coherence, as well as higher psychological well-being and lower depressive symptoms. These results are useful for general theoretical and methodological reflection, as well as for their specific bearing on our project. First, our scale has proven to be a valid tool for assessing self-efficacy of patients with a relapsing–remitting form of the disease and with a moderate disability. These are people who face unpredictable symptoms and a fluctuating course of their disease, but who are generally autonomous and must cope with daily work, family, and social commitments. Our scale is therefore suitable for patients with these characteristics, for whom the two considered dimensions of self-efficacy (goal setting and symptom management) are crucial. Second, the results – confirming the links between self-efficacy, sense of coherence, psychological well-being and depressive symptoms – go in the same direction that emerged from the in-depth study discussed in the sub-section titled: *The role of identity, sense of coherence and self-efficacy for the adjustment to illness* which further substantiates the validity of our theoretical model (see Chapters 1 and 2). Finally, as discussed in *The Pilot Project,* this measure of self-efficacy was proved suitable for capturing a short-term intervention effect: we recall that at the conclusion of the four sessions patients reported greater self-efficacy in their disease management than the comparison group. In relation to the continuation of our activities, the combination of these results led us to maintain the scale, without modification, in the questionnaire used (*Me and my life*, Appendix 4) for the project dedicated to newly diagnosed patients and to conduct further investigations into the role of self-efficacy among young adults in the early years of the disease, the results of which will be presented in the section *Identity and MS: The double challenge of newly diagnosed young adults.*

The project for newly diagnosed patients

As anticipated, based on the experience of the pilot project, we have implemented a specific intervention program for newly diagnosed people, which has also been evaluated. Recalling, the intervention consists of five sessions, plus a continuation and reminder session (follow-up) after six months and a final in-depth session (focus group) after one year, the modalities and contents of which are presented in Chapter 3.

To evaluate the effectiveness of the intervention project, we compared the responses to the *Me and my life* questionnaire described above (see Figure 4.5) from two groups of newly diagnosed patients with similar characteristics (in terms of age, gender, years since diagnosis), but with one fundamental difference: whether or not they had participated in the intervention. One group consisted of 54 people who had participated in the project sessions (intervention group), the other group of 31 people who had not participated in the project sessions (comparison group). The aim was to compare the responses of the two patient groups to the same questionnaire over time. The newly diagnosed patients who participated in the intervention were between 21 and 65 years old (with a mean of 38 years, standard deviation 12 years); 61% were women, and the average duration of illness was one and a

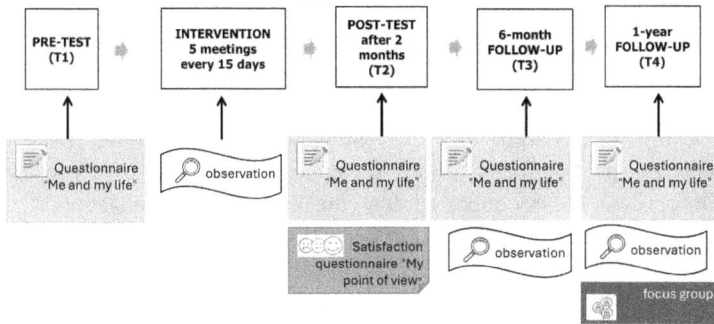

Figure 4.5 The project for newly diagnosed patients: Timing and measurement tools.

half years. The newly diagnosed patients in the comparison group were between 20 and 63 years old (with a mean of 35 years, standard deviation 12 years), 55% were women, and the mean disease duration was 1.8 years (for details of the study, see Calandri et al., 2017a). The assessment of satisfaction with the experience was, of course, conducted only among the participants of the sessions, using the instruments already presented above (the *My point of view* questionnaire, the focus group and the observation; see Figure 4.5), with the exception of the audio-recording of the sessions (see Figure 4.1).

The intervention for newly diagnosed patients was characterized by a high and constant participation: 80% of the participating patients followed the entire course and 67% were present at the last session after one year. In terms of satisfaction of the intervention, almost all patients (93%) expressed a positive or very positive evaluation of the experience, 74% rated it as helpful or very helpful, 98% would repeat or recommend the experience to other patients, and 65% reported a positive change in their feelings and attitudes.

During the focus groups, one year after the last session of the intervention, patients recognized and emphasized the importance of the psychological support function that the sessions had in such an overwhelming time after diagnosis. The group recognized what a fundamental opportunity it was for them to encounter with others, which required for some to overcome their fear of comparison with other patients who may be at a more advanced stage of the disease and thus represented their possible, feared future conditions. In the focus groups, patients also emphasized the benefits of the group sessions in terms of the practical impact on their daily lives; this applies to learning relaxation techniques that were practiced during the sessions and then became part of participants' daily lives whenever they felt the need to relax, such as in the case of a medical examination.

Hence, many patients expressed a desire to continue the sessions over time and make them part of the treatment of their illness. Among the positive and unforeseen effects of the intervention, the creation of new social bonds was felt; friendships were formed between group participants that lasted beyond the duration of the intervention (see Box 4.7).

Box 4.7   The participants' words. Some considerations from the focus groups of the project for newly diagnosed patients

The following are some examples of phrases said by newly diagnosed patients during the focus groups conducted at the end of the cycle of group sessions. Many reported that the meetings offered support after diagnosis.

The meetings are useful right away to deal with the diagnosis, then later for support... (woman, youth group 20-35 years old).

At the time of diagnosis, they give you a lot of medical information, but psychologically there is little support (woman, adult group 36-50 years old).

It was very helpful to meet with the neurologist (man, adult group 36-50 years old).

I got a great benefit from these meetings, because I learned about the illness (man, adult group over 50 years old).

Relaxation and breathing were very helpful (man, youth group 20-35 years old).

I used breathing when I had to have an MRI (woman, adult group 36-50 years old).

Many participants appreciated the venue of the meetings:

It's good to have the meetings here [at the Castle], outside the hospital... it's a nice place, in the hospital it would be more comfortable, but it's not so nice... it's sadder (woman, youth group 20-35 years old)

Many emphasized the importance of comparison with others:

Sharing with others helps to move forward, it helps me to get unstuck, I talk about the disease with fewer problems (woman, youth group 20-35 years old).

The best thing was the comparison... with others you think more positively (man, adult group 36-50 years old).

Considerations emerged from some patients about the experience of the group and the usefulness of continuing it over time.

At first you don't know who you might meet, what stage of the disease they are at, and that scares you a little. But seeing that other participants are like you, it calms you down (man, adult group 36-50 years old).

It was a bit tiring, but this way you told it, you told yourself too... it weighs but it frees you... in other contexts you can talk about it but it's different... (woman, youth group 20-35 years old).

It would be useful to continue the meetings over time, even contrasting with people of different ages (woman, youth group 20-35 years old).

As for the evaluation of effectiveness, which was carried out using the *Me and my life* questionnaire, the patients who participated in the groups reported a better quality of life and a higher level of optimism one year after the intervention. In addition, depressive symptoms decreased between the start of the intervention and the six-month follow-up and tended to remain constant thereafter. Affective well-being also increased six months after the intervention and showed a tendency toward stability over time. Overall, the results are consistent with those of the pilot project. In addition, the positive effects of the intervention remain after one year, not only in terms of reducing symptoms, but also in terms of promoting positive aspects, particularly in relation to optimism (Figure 4.6).

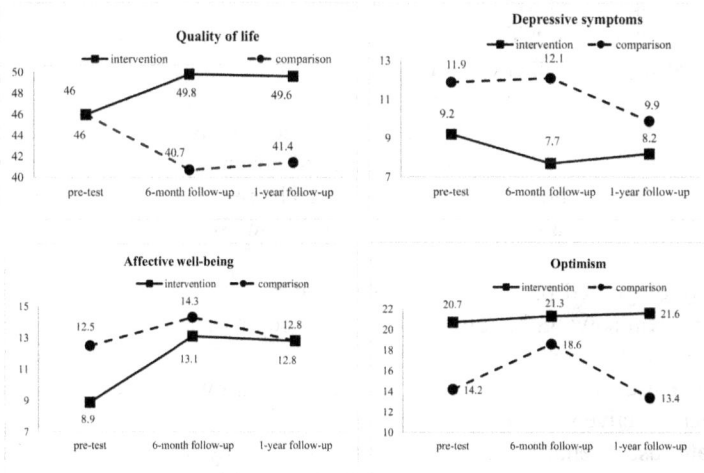

Figure 4.6 Evaluation of intervention effectiveness for newly diagnosed patients (mean scores of quality of life, depressive symptoms, affective well-being and optimism in the intervention group and in the comparison group).

The role of coping strategies and sense of coherence for the adjustment to illness in newly diagnosed patients

The data collected during the pilot project showed that a greater sense of coherence was associated with a better quality of life and greater affective well-being, as well as less depressive symptoms (see the section *The role of identity, sense of coherence and self-efficacy for the adjustment to illness*). The analysis of data collected from newly diagnosed patients confirmed the associations between the sense of coherence and the three aspects of adjustment considered, confirming the central importance of this dimension also in the first years of the illness (Calandri et al., 2018). As sense of coherence is one of the central constructs of our theoretical model, we wanted to investigate the role it plays in newly diagnosed patients, especially in relation to coping strategies (problem solving, emotion-centered coping, avoidance-centered coping; see Box 4.1).

The use of coping strategies in people with MS is an aspect that has received increasing attention in recent years, but there are few studies on newly diagnosed patients. Early work on coping in MS patients has shown that, in general, problem-solving strategies are the most adaptive way of coping with illness, while emotional coping and avoidance are dysfunctional (McCabe, 2006; Pakenham, 1999; Rabinowitz & Arnett, 2009). However, recent studies suggest that both emotional coping and avoidance may play a positive role in adjustment to MS. Especially in the short term, both strategies appear to be more useful than problem solving for coping with symptoms and events that are difficult to control, for dispelling negative thoughts about disease progression, and for expressing and sharing one's emotional experiences (Dennison et al., 2010; Mikula et al., 2015; Pakenham, 2006; Roubinov et al., 2015). As studies have reported conflicting results on the role of emotional coping and avoidance in the early years of the illness (Bianchi et al., 2014; Lode et al., 2009; Tan-Kristanto & Kiropoulos, 2015), we decided to investigate these aspects further by examining the role of coping strategies in adaptation to one's illness and the possible mediating role of sense of coherence between coping and adaptation. Our hypothesis suggested that coping style could influence the representation of life as having a sense of coherence and that this would affect well-being and the discomfort experienced by people (for details, see Calandri et al., 2017b). The main results are presented below (see Figure 4.7):

- Newly diagnosed patients who make greater use of strategies not only based on problem solving, but also on emotional coping and avoidance report better adjustment to illness.
- Greater use of problem solving is accompanied by better quality of life and higher affective well-being.
- Greater use of emotional coping is accompanied by the perception of a higher sense of coherence and this in turn reduces depressive symptoms.
- Greater use of avoidance is accompanied by the perception of a higher sense of coherence and this in turn reduces depressive symptoms, as well as promoting quality of life and affective well-being.

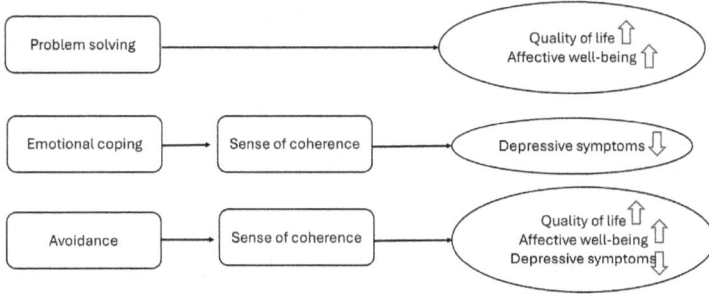

Figure 4.7 Relationships between coping strategies (problem solving, emotional coping and avoidance), sense of coherence, and adjustment to illness (quality of life, depressive symptoms and affective well-being).

Our results thus illustrate that even coping strategies that are normally considered less adaptive (emotional coping and avoidance) can play a positive role in the first years after diagnosis, as they have an impact on the sense of coherence. First, the ability to express emotions and share them with others seems to be a useful strategy to reduce depressive experiences. Expressing emotions can help patients understand their feelings and cope with their experiences, which strengthens the sense of coherence, which in turn reduces depressive symptoms.

Avoidance can also be an adaptive way of coping, at least in the short term, with symptoms that are difficult to control and change, and the unpredictability of the course of the illness. This strategy can be a way of avoiding what cannot be controlled and can thus increase the perceived sense of coherence, which in turn has a positive effect on adjustment, provided it does not become the usual coping strategy.

These results lead us to some reflections, both from a theoretical point of view and in terms of intervention. We know that the post-diagnosis period can be characterized by strong emotions, angry reactions, anxiety, and depression. It is a time when people learn to cope with a new condition that is hardly controllable and/or predictable. Different coping strategies may prove helpful, but a central role is always played by the ability to give a sense of coherence to the experience one is having, to understand what is going on, to feel that one has the resources to cope with the situation and to find meaning in what one is experiencing. From a psychological intervention perspective, it is useful to promote strategies based on problem solving to help people set realistic and meaningful goals for themselves in a state of illness that imposes severe limitations and undermines the realization of pre-diagnosis plans. The ability to deal with emotions also needs to be strengthened, especially to counteract depressive symptoms. Finally, avoidance should also be accepted in the initial period after diagnosis and can be recognized as a functional strategy to reduce, for example, the feeling of helplessness that the patient often experiences and the resulting depressive reactions. However, it is a coping strategy that is useful in the short term for certain situations and should be considered a prerequisite for setting more adaptive and realistic goals. Therefore, different coping strategies must be strengthened by taking into account the complexity of the factors influencing adjustment to one's illness, particularly the amount of time that has elapsed since diagnosis. Our findings clearly highlight the importance for professionals working with MS patients to help them regain a sense of coherence in their life with the illness.

Identity and MS: The double challenge of newly diagnosed young adults

In recent years, an important part of our research has focused on adaptation to the disease in young adults (18–35 years), who are the majority of newly diagnosed patients. As outlined in Chapter 2, young adulthood represents a life stage in which the individual has to cope with several developmental tasks, including redefining relationships with the family of origin, achieving progressive autonomy not only economically but also emotionally, making educational and career decisions, entering into an intimate emotional relationship and deciding to become a parent or not. A diagnosis of illness in young adulthood represents a profound break in the individual life cycle that necessitates a process of redefining one's own identity. In particular, one must face the "double challenge" of redefining one's identity as a young adult and as a person suffering from a chronic illness.

Data from questionnaires completed by newly diagnosed young adult patients showed that they report fewer disabling symptoms and better physical health compared to newly diagnosed patients of older age groups, as already reported in the literature (Jones et al., 2012). Although the newly diagnosed young adults in our sample do not report a particularly critical situation from a purely physical perspective, they do report significant depressive symptoms and lower levels of affective well-being and quality of life than the healthy population, findings that are again consistent with the literature (Buchanan et al., 2010; Rainone et al., 2017; Solari et al., 1999). As had already emerged from the data of the pilot project, also among newly diagnosed young adult patients the redefinition of identity, central especially at this age, plays a key role with respect to the adjustment to the illness. Specifically, greater identity satisfaction is not only linked to fewer depressive symptoms, but also to higher levels of optimism and affective well-being. Precisely with respect to affective well-being, the role of self-efficacy in MS management is confirmed among newly diagnosed young adult patients (Calandri et al., 2018).

Starting from these findings, a specific part of our research work focused on a more in-depth analysis of the role of identity and self-efficacy with respect to depressive symptoms and affective well-being among newly diagnosed young adults. In particular, we wanted to investigate whether identity satisfaction has an influence on perceived self-efficacy in disease management (in the two components of goal setting and symptom management) and whether this, in turn, affects the depressive symptoms and well-being experienced (for details see Calandri et al., 2019).

The results show that patients who report greater satisfaction with their identity report:

- fewer depressive symptoms;
- greater self-efficacy in goal setting, which in turn is linked to a greater positive affect and
- greater self-efficacy in symptom management, which in turn is linked to a lower negative affect.

The relationships between the variables are illustrated in Figure 4.8.

In other words, identity appears to have a direct effect on depressive symptoms, with people who are more satisfied with their identity having fewer depressive symptoms. In addition, identity has an indirect effect on affective well-being through the mediation of perceived self-efficacy. In particular, the two components of self-efficacy (the ability to set meaningful goals and the ability to manage symptoms) have different effects upon one's self-image and self-experience, with the former affecting positive feelings and the latter negative feelings. Especially, the ability to set meaningful goals is associated with greater positive affect, while the ability to cope with symptoms is associated with lower negative affect.

The results obtained have significant implications, both from a theoretical perspective and for interventions. Identity and self-efficacy are confirmed as two closely related constructs that play a central role in one's adjustment to their illness in the first years after diagnosis. Identity satisfaction appears to play a particularly important role in protecting against depressive symptoms. Young adults who manage to redefine their identity and develop a new self-image that includes chronic illness are less likely to suffer from depression. Identity also has an indirect effect on well-being through self-efficacy, feeling capable of coping with one's illness in everyday life appears to be a crucial dimension for experiencing greater emotional well-being. In particular, young people who feel more able to set meaningful goals for themselves experience positive feelings and feel active and determined.

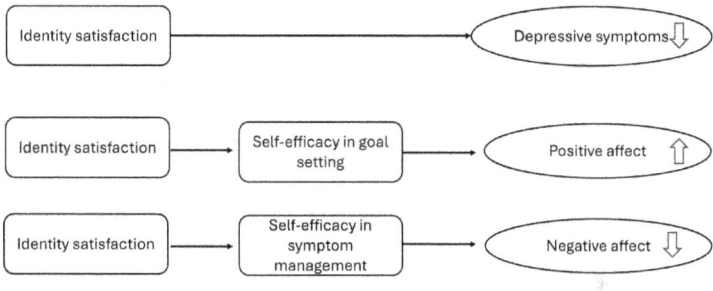

Figure 4.8 Relationships between identity satisfaction, self-efficacy in dealing with MS (goal setting and symptom management), depressive symptoms and affective well-being (positive affect and negative affect).

At the same time, young people who see themselves as better able to manage the numerous and often uncontrollable symptoms of illness experience fewer negative emotional experiences (e.g., fear, anxiety, pessimism).

From the point of view of intervention, these results emphasize the need to act on both identity and self-efficacy, considering the close relationship between the two constructs. Redefining identity and life goals, not only in relation to the developmental tasks of young adulthood, but also in relation to the limits and possibilities of one's illness, thus appears crucial to protecting against malaise and to actively promote the well-being of newly diagnosed young adults.

Identity and newly diagnosed young adults: A comparison with healthy peers

The centrality of the construct of identity for young adults prompted us to further deepen our understanding of the role it plays in adjustment to illness in the early years following diagnosis. For this reason, part of our research focuses on examining the roles that various aspects of identity satisfaction play in the experience of well-being and discomfort, in newly diagnosed young adults and in young adults who do not suffer from a chronic illness. Specifically, we chose to compare two groups of young adults (one with and one without MS) to better understand the specificities of the transition to adulthood for young people with this disease and to investigate whether and to what identity satisfaction plays a different role in the two groups (for details, see Calandri et al., 2020).

As illustrated in Box 4.1, the identity construct we studied includes varying aspects defined as "identity motives" (Vignoles, 2011; Vignoles et al., 2006; we mention them briefly: self-esteem, efficacy, continuity, belongingness, distinctiveness and meaning). Some of these are particularly threatened when a young adult is diagnosed with MS. Considering the disease undermines: efficacy, as the symptoms and disability negatively affect the sense of control over events; continuity, as a gap is created between "before" and "after" the diagnosis; and meaning, as the unpredictability and multiple symptoms threaten the perception of the meaning of one's life. Our aim is to investigate whether differing identity motives play a different role in depressive symptoms and quality of life between young adults with MS and healthy young adults. The results showed that:

- greater endorsement of the meaning motive is associated with fewer depressive symptoms among young people with MS;
- greater endorsement of distinctiveness tends to be associated with greater depressive symptoms among young people with MS, whereas greater distinctiveness is associated with fewer depressive symptoms among healthy young people and
- less endorsement of continuity and belonging are associated with poorer quality of life among young people with MS.

The results are summarized in Figure 4.9.

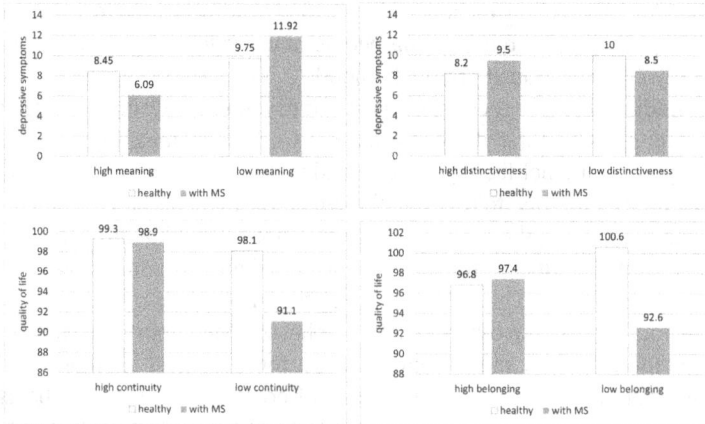

Figure 4.9 Mean scores of depressive symptoms and quality of life among youth with MS and healthy youth in relation to identity motives (meaning, distinctiveness, continuity, belonging).

In other words, the perception of meaning seems to be particularly important for young patients to protect them from the risk of developing depressive symptoms, whereas this relationship is more nuanced in healthy young people. The illness thus confirms itself as a situation of identity threat that profoundly affects the perception of the meaning of life. The illness also represents a major break between "before" and "after" the diagnosis, thus threatening the sense of continuity in one's life experience. In the human life cycle, young adulthood is usually a period of discontinuity characterized by normative changes in different areas of life (work, family, friendships, emotional relationships), but in the case of a young adult diagnosed with MS, it seems to be especially important to re-establish a sense of continuity in one's life in order to cope with the unforeseen manifestations of the one's illness. This could be the reason why the perception of continuity is most important for a good quality of life in young people with chronic illness. Maintaining a sense of closeness to other people was also identified as a factor in quality of life, especially in young people with MS. This could be related to the need for social support, notably important resource in coping with the difficulties associated with chronic illness. Furthermore, the feeling of being accepted by others can counteract the feelings of exclusion or fear of social stigmatization that often characterize the experience of people with a chronic illness and that have a profound impact on their quality of life.

Ultimately, the fact that distinctiveness protects healthy young people from feelings of depression, but not young people with MS, suggests that for healthy young people, feeling unique and different from others may be helpful for positive self-definition, whereas for young people with the disease, the perception of difference may be conditioned by the illness itself. The perception of being different increases feelings of isolation and stigmatization, which can lead to depression. This result substantiates that a young person with MS feels the need above all to perceive themselves as "equal" to other young people in order to reduce the discomfort of their already complex transition to adulthood.

These findings offer suggestions relating to psychological support for newly diagnosed young adults. First, the importance of working on meaning is emphasized, particularly to counteract feelings of depression. Second, it is imperative to reflect on the need for continuity, to reweave the thread of life experience and to keep the "before" and "after" of the diagnosis together, not by ruminating about what one can no longer do because of the illness, but by redefining plans of action according to real possibilities. Third, underscoring the importance of feeling a sense of belonging and closeness to others clearly emphasizes the importance of working on effective communication and the ability to ask for help. Last, a broader reflection on the importance of feeling "the same" or "different" from peers may be useful to counteract the depressive experiences that young patients often have.

MS in women: Identity and the role of motherhood in newly diagnosed women

In recent years, in addition to the experiences of newly diagnosed young adults, a considerable amount of our research has focused on the experience of illness in newly diagnosed women, particularly in relation to their role as mothers. As described earlier, women are more affected by MS at a stage in their lives when many are considering motherhood or are already engaged in childcare. Some decide to have a child only after diagnosis, others have young children at the time of diagnosis and others have school-age children or already teenagers or young adults still living at home. In all of these cases, parenting can be an additional physical and psychological strain above that associated with chronic illness. The symptoms of MS can interfere with the fulfillment of the parental role, especially when one's children are young; we are thinking primarily of fatigue, but also of coping with relapses and the side effects of therapies. In addition, concerns about the unpredictability of one's illness also represent an emotional burden that can make it strenuous to care for children of all ages. All in all, such physical and psychological struggles can worsen the quality of life and exacerbate patients' anxiety and depression. In countries where housework and childcare are still predominantly the responsibility of women, these effects of parenting-related illnesses are particularly evident in patients. There is also the important issue of pregnancy.

Until a few years ago, the "multiple sclerosis – motherhood" binomial was hardly considered, as the disease was seen as a condition that was incompatible with motherhood and pregnancy, and consequently, it was discouraged. Today, this is no longer the case and many women are faced with a difficult decision in this regard.

Researchers' interest in MS in relation to the experience of motherhood is therefore new, and it is only in recent years that studies have been published on the subject. In parallel with the increase in medical knowledge about pregnancy with a MS diagnosis, psychological studies have focused on maternity choices following diagnosis and the psychological experiences of mothers in the postpartum period (Kosmala-Anderson & Wallace, 2013; Payne & McPherson, 2010; Prunty et al., 2008). Only in recent years have studies taken an interest in the broader experiences of mothers with MS and the issue of balancing parental responsibilities and disease management during their children's growing years, from infancy to adolescence (Willson et al., 2018). Although interest in these issues is currently gradually increasing, the topic is still under-researched from a scientific and psychological perspective.

Based on these considerations, in our work we want to investigate the topic of maternal function in women with MS. To this end, we compared women with and without children in terms of adjustment to the illness and studied the specific role of identity satisfaction in adjustment to MS in these two groups. The focus of our interest on identity is motivated by the central role that this aspect plays in both adaptation to MS and parental functioning.

This in-depth study was conducted with a subgroup of 74 newly diagnosed women (32 of whom were mothers) aged between 19 and 57 years (average age 38 years). All mothers in our sample had children prior to diagnosis; most of them had only one child who was between 2 and 17 years old at the time of the study, but there were also those who already had adult children and lived with them in the same household (for details, see Graziano et al., 2020). The results showed that:

- Mothers report greater depressive symptoms, lower affective well-being and lower identity satisfaction than childless women, and these differences tend to increase as time passes from the moment of diagnosis.
- Identity satisfaction emerges as important for adjustment to illness, particularly for mothers, with lower identity satisfaction associated with greater depressive symptoms and lower affective well-being in mothers than in childless women.

The results are shown in Figure 4.10.

The greater depressive symptoms and lower well-being reported by mothers are likely related to the burden of the parenting role and the physical and emotional distress of the illness. Thus, these symptoms contribute to the concern that one's illness may impair their ability to fulfill the parenting role and negatively affect their

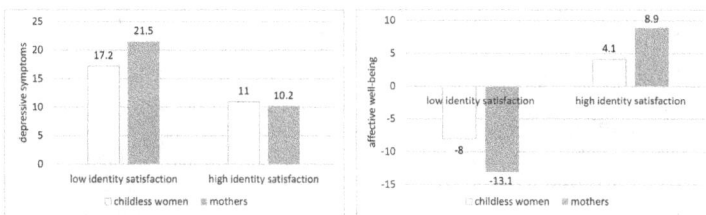

Figure 4.10 Mean scores of depressive symptoms and affective well-being among mothers and childless women in relation to identity satisfaction.

children or child. The differences between mothers and childless women become more pronounced as years pass after diagnosis, which is likely a sign of difficulties that increase over time. In particular, it is likely that childless women manage to achieve a relatively stable psychological equilibrium over time, whereas mothers must constantly redefine their role in relation to the needs and demands of their children, which change as the children develop. It is precisely this ability to re-define one's own identity that appears to be central to adapting to MS in the early years of the illness, especially for mothers. Indeed, women with a parental role face the double challenge of redefining their identity as a mother and as a person with a chronic illness. Mothers who are better able to cope with this dual challenge appear to adapt better to their illness, characterized not only by fewer depressive symptoms but also by a greater sense of well-being.

These findings have important implications for designing psychological support for women with MS, while emphasizing the special attention that needs to be given to women with children. Promoting a redefinition of the identity of mothers with MS means, above all, improving their ability to perceive their role as a parent, taking into account the limitations and possibilities of their illness, as well as scrupulously managing pressing concerns about their own future and that of their children. In addition to promoting self-efficacy and coping with one's own emotions, work also focused on how communication can prove to be central in making it easier for mothers to seek help and activate social support networks, starting with those close to them (one's partner, extended family, circle of friends) as well as requesting information and seeking support from specific professionals (neurologist, gynecologist, psychologist).

The results reported in this chapter demonstrate the essential role of research in our project. Research links theory and intervention in a circular process in which the intervention is structured from the theoretical basis and new theoretical considerations are developed from the data collected through the intervention. The results we presented confirm the validity of our proposed intervention to promote adjustment to chronic illness in the first years after diagnosis. In addition, the data we collected allowed us to conduct more in-depth targeted studies on the constructs that form the cornerstone of our theoretical model. Particularly, the findings presented in this section regarding young adults and mothers have led us to develop new directions of intervention and research that we will present in the following chapter.

References

Airlie, J., Baker, G. A., Smith, S. J., & Young, C. A. (2001). Measuring the impact of multiple sclerosis on psychosocial functioning: The development of a new self-efficacy scale. *Clinical Rehabilitation, 15*(3), 259–265.

Andresen, E. M., Malmgren, J. A., Carter, W. B., & Patrick, D. L. (1994). Screening for depression in well older adults: Evaluation of a short form of the CES-D (Center for Epidemiologic Studies Depression Scale). *American Journal of Preventive Medicine, 10*, 77–84.

Antonovsky, A. (1993). The structure and properties of the sense of coherence scale. *Social Science and Medicine, 36*, 725–733.

Bianchi, V., De Giglio, L., Prosperini, L., Mancinelli, C., De Angelis, F., Barletta, V., & Pozzilli, C. (2014). Mood and coping in clinically isolated syndrome and multiple sclerosis. *Acta Neurologica Scandinavica, 129*(6), 374–381.

Bonino, S. (2021). *Coping with chronic illness. Theories, issues and lived experiences.* Routledge.

Bonino, S., Graziano, F., Borghi, M., Marengo, D., Molinengo, G., & Calandri, E. (2018). The self-efficacy in multiple sclerosis (SEMS) scale: Development and validation with Rasch analysis. *European Journal of Psychological Assessment, 34*, 352–360.

Borghi, M., Bonino, S., Graziano, F., & Calandri, E. (2018). Exploring change in a group-based psychological intervention for multiple sclerosis patients. *Disability and Rehabilitation, 40*, 1671–1678.

Buchanan, R. J., Minden, S. L., Chakravorty, B. J., Hatcher, W., Tyry, T., & Vollmer, T. (2010). A pilot study of young adults with multiple sclerosis: Demographic, disease, treatment, and psychosocial characteristics. *Disability and Health Journal, 3*, 262–270.

Calandri, E., Graziano, F., Borghi, M., & Bonino, S. (2017a). Improving the quality of life and psychological well-being of recently diagnosed multiple sclerosis patients: Preliminary evaluation of a group-based cognitive behavioral intervention. *Disability and Rehabilitation, 39*, 1474–1481.

Calandri, E., Graziano, F., Borghi, M., & Bonino, S. (2017b). Coping strategies and adjustment to multiple sclerosis among recently diagnosed patients: The mediating role of sense of coherence. *Clinical Rehabilitation, 31*, 1386–1395.

Calandri, E., Graziano, F., Borghi, M., & Bonino, S. (2018). Depression, positive and negative affect, optimism and health-related quality of life in recently diagnosed multiple sclerosis patients: The role of identity, sense of coherence, and self-efficacy. *Journal of Happiness Studies, 19*, 277–295.

Calandri, E., Graziano, F., Borghi, M., & Bonino, S. (2019). Young adults' adjustment to a recent diagnosis of multiple sclerosis: The role of identity satisfaction and self-efficacy. *Disability and Health Journal, 12*, 72–78.

Calandri, E., Graziano, F., Borghi, M., Bonino, S., & Cattelino, E. (2020). The role of identity motives on quality of life and depressive symptoms: A comparison between young adults with multiple sclerosis and healthy peers. *Frontiers in Psychology, Developmental Psychology Section, 11*, Article, 589815.

Chiesi, F., Galli, S., Primi, C., Innocenti Borgi, P., & Bonacchi, A. (2013). The accuracy of the Life Orientation Test-Revised (LOT-R) in measuring dispositional optimism: Evidence from item response theory analyses. *Journal of Personality Assessment, 95*, 523–529.

Dennison, L., Moss-Morris, R., Silber, E., Galea, I., & Chalder, T. (2010). Cognitive and behavioural correlates of different domains of psychological adjustment in early-stage multiple sclerosis. *Journal of Psychosomatic Research, 69*, 353–361.

Fava, G. A. (1983). Assessing depressive symptoms across cultures: Italian validation of the CES-D self-rating scale. *Journal of Clinical Psychology, 39*, 249–251.

Graziano, F., Calandri, E., Borghi, M., & Bonino, S. (2014). The effects of a group-based cognitive behavioral therapy on people with multiple sclerosis: A randomized controlled trial. *Clinical Rehabilitation, 28*, 264–274.

Graziano, F., Calandri, E., Borghi, M., & Bonino, S. (2020). Adjustment to multiple sclerosis and identity satisfaction among newly diagnosed women: What role does motherhood play? *Women and Health, 60*, 271–283.

Jones, K. H., Ford, D. V., Jones, P. A., John, A., Middleton, R. M., Lockhart-Jones, H., Osborne, L. A., & Noble, J. G. (2012). A large-scale study of anxiety and depression in people with multiple sclerosis: A survey via the web portal of the UK MS register. *PLoS ONE, 7*, 1–10.

Klevan, G., Jacobsen, C. O., Aarseth, J. H., Myhr, K. M., Nyland, H., Glad, S., Lode, K., Figved, N., Larsen, J. P., & Farbu, E. (2014). Health related quality of life in patients recently diagnosed with multiple sclerosis. *Acta Neurologica Scandinavica, 129*, 21–26.

Kosmala-Anderson, J., & Wallace, L. M. (2013). A qualitative study of the childbearing experience of women living with multiple sclerosis. *Disability and Rehabilitation, 35,* 976–981.

Lode, K., Bru, E., Klevan, G., Myhr, K. M., Nyland, H., & Larsen, J. P. (2009). Depressive symptoms and coping in newly diagnosed patients with multiple sclerosis. *Multiple Sclerosis, 15,* 638–643.

Manzi, C., Vignoles, V. L., & Regalia, C. (2010). Accommodating a new identity: Possible selves, identity change and well-being across two life-transitions. *European Journal of Social Psychology, 40,* 970–984.

McCabe, M. (2006). A longitudinal study of coping strategies and quality of life among people with multiple sclerosis. *Journal of Clinical Psychology in Medical Settings, 13,* 367–377.

McCabe, M. P., & McKern, S. (2002). Quality of life and multiple sclerosis: Comparison between people with multiple sclerosis and people from the general population. *Journal of Clinical Psychology in Medical Settings, 9,* 287–295.

Mikula, P., Nagyova, I., Krokavcova, M., Vitkova, M., Rosenberger, J., Szilasiova, J., Gdovinova, Z., Groothoff, J. W., & Van Dijk, J. P. (2015). The mediating effect of coping on the association between fatigue and quality of life in patients with multiple sclerosis. *Psychology, Health and Medicine, 20,* 653–661.

Pakenham, K. I. (1999). Adjustment to multiple sclerosis: Application of a stress and coping model. *Health Psychology, 18,* 383–392.

Pakenham, K. I. (2001). Coping with multiple sclerosis: Development of a measure. *Psychology, Health and Medicine, 6,* 411–428.

Pakenham, K. I. (2006). Investigation of the coping antecedents to positive outcomes and distress in multiple sclerosis (MS). *Psychology and Health, 21,* 633–649.

Payne, D., & McPherson, K. (2010). Becoming mothers. Multiple sclerosis and motherhood: A qualitative study. *Disability and Rehabilitation, 32,* 629–638.

Peres, D. S., Rodrigues, P., Viero, F. T., Frare, J. M., Kudsi, S. Q., Meira, G. M., & Trevisan, G. (2022). Prevalence of depression and anxiety in the different clinical forms of multiple sclerosis and associations with disability: A systematic review and meta-analysis. *Brain, Behavior, & Immunity-Health, 24,* 100484.

Prunty, M., Sharpe, L., Butow, P., & Fulcher, G. (2008). The motherhood choice: Themes arising in the decision-making process for women with multiple sclerosis. *Multiple Sclerosis, 14,* 701–704.

Rabinowitz, A. R., & Arnett, P. A. (2009). A longitudinal analysis of cognitive dysfunction, coping, and depression in multiple sclerosis. *Neuropsychology, 23,* 581–591.

Rainone, N., Chiodi, A., Lanzillo, R., Magri, V., Napolitano, A., Morra, V. B., Valerio, P., & Freda, M. F. (2017). Affective disorders and Health-Related Quality of Life (HRQoL) in adolescents and young adults with Multiple Sclerosis (MS): The moderating role of resilience. *Quality of Life Research, 26,* 727–736.

Rigby, S. A., Domenech, C., Thornton, E. W., Tedman, S., & Young, C. A. (2003). Development and validation of a self-efficacy measure for people with multiple sclerosis: The multiple sclerosis self-efficacy scale. *Multiple Sclerosis, 9,* 73–81.

Roubinov, D. S., Turner, A. P., & Williams, R. M. (2015). Coping among individuals with multiple sclerosis: Evaluating a goodness-of-fit model. *Rehabilitation Psychology, 60,* 162–168.

Scheier, M. F., Carver, C. S., & Bridges, M. W. (1994). Distinguishing optimism from neuroticism (and trait anxiety, self-mastery and self-esteem): A re-evaluation of the Life Orientation Test. *Journal of Personality and Social Psychology, 67,* 1063–1078.

Schwartz, C. E., Coulthard-Morris, L., Zeng, Q., & Retzlaff, P. (1996). Measuring self-efficacy in people with multiple sclerosis: A validation study. *Archives of Physical Medicine and Rehabilitation, 77,* 394–398.

Solari, A., Filippini, G., Mendozzi, L., Ghezzi, A., Cifani, S., Barbieri, E., Baldini, S., Salmaggi, A., La Mantia, L., Farinotti, M., Caputo, D., & Mosconi, P. (1999). Validation of

Italian multiple sclerosis quality of life 54 questionnaire. *Journal of Neurology, Neurosurgery & Psychiatry, 67*, 158–162.

Tan-Kristanto, S., & Kiropoulos, L. A. (2015). Resilience, self-efficacy, coping styles and depressive and anxiety symptoms in those newly diagnosed with multiple sclerosis. *Psychology, Health and Medicine, 20*, 635–645.

Terracciano, A., McCrae, R. R., & Costa, P. (2003). Factorial and construct validity of the Italian Positive and Negative Affect Schedule (PANAS). *European Journal of Psychological Assessment, 19*, 131–141.

Vignoles, V. L. (2011). Identity motives. In K. Luycke, S. J. Schwartz, & V. L. Vignoles (Eds.), *Handbook of identity theory and research* (pp. 403–432). Springer.

Vignoles, V. L., Regalia, C., Manzi, C., Golledge, J., & Scabini, E. (2006). Beyond self-esteem: Influence of multiple motives on identity construction. *Journal of Personality and Social Psychology, 90*, 308–333.

Ware, J. E., Keller, S. D., & Kosinski, M. (1995). *SF-12: How to score the SF-12 physical and mental health summary scales*. Health Institute, New England Medical Center.

Watson, D., Clark, L. A., & Tellegen, A. (1988). Development and validation of brief measures of positive and negative affect: The PANAS scales. *Journal of Personality and Social Psychology, 54*, 1063–1070.

Willson, C. L., Tetley, J., Lloyd, C., Messmer Uccelli, M., & MacKian, S. (2018). The impact of multiple sclerosis on the identity of mothers in Italy. *Disability and Rehabilitation, 40*, 1456–1467.

5 Beyond the individual

Multiple sclerosis and parent–child relationships

Federica Graziano, Emanuela Calandri and Martina Borghi

Introduction

Over the course of these years, our clinical experience conducted with the various participants in the groups has highlighted the importance of family relationships: as a matter of fact, the issue of an individual's adjustment to multiple sclerosis (MS) cannot be separated from their embedded familial relationships.

As was extensively discussed in Chapter 3, during group meetings, participants are asked to reflect on the area of family relationships in relation to their experience of illness. For example, when they are asked to reflect on redefining life goals and strategies for achieving them, or when discussing effective communication, inevitably family relationships are one of the primary aspects addressed. Beyond the facilitator's invitation to reflect on these aspects, the topic of family relationships is recognized by all as extremely relevant. Participants in the groups are children, sometimes partners or parents, and their experiences in their various family roles are inevitably intertwined with the challenges posed by MS and the resources through which to cope with the illness.

Not only our clinical experience with groups, but also some of our research findings have contributed to highlight the role of family relationships with respect to illness. As illustrated in Chapter 4, our research also explored some aspects of the experience of women with MS through a comparison between mothers and childless women, highlighting how the experience of the illness must inevitably be considered in relation to parenthood.

Building on these considerations over time, the horizon of our clinical and research work has gradually broadened, and we have developed new directions of intervention and research focused on the topic of MS and parent–child relationships.

Upon one aspect, we focused on young adults who represent most newly diagnosed MS patients and who, not only in the Italian context, often still live in their family of origin. The diagnosis of MS poses a challenge not only for them but for the entire family system in which they are embedded, and often their parents do not know how to cope with it. In our clinical experience, we have frequently encountered young adult patients who experience relationship difficulties with their parents and sometimes parents who ask for support in managing their role.

DOI: 10.4324/9781003484400-5

In another aspect, we've devoted ourselves to investigating the experience of parents with MS, a dimension still little addressed in psychological literature. Again, in our clinical experience with groups, we often encountered parents expressing their difficulties, particularly in communicating this illness to their children, or in reconciling their parental role with the symptoms of the illness especially when they have young children.

Considering the relevance of these topics, therefore, we felt it was important to close our book with this last chapter, focused on both parenting young adult children with MS and being parents (mothers and fathers) with MS. After a brief theoretical introduction, we will present some research findings and operational directions for supportive psychological interventions targeting both parents who have young adult children with MS and parents with MS who must cope with parental tasks while reconciling with the burden of their illness.

MS as a challenge for the family system (Federica Graziano)

In recent years, scientific literature has examined the psychological aspects of MS, broadening its gaze from the patient's experience to the experience of the entire system of relationships in which one is a part of with specific attention to their immediate and extended family system. The disease, in fact, does not only concern the individual but has profound repercussions on the experiences of all family members. With a very effective expression, some authors state that MS is a "family matter" (Boström & Nilsagård, 2016), suggesting it is not an exaggeration to say that each family member is affected by the disease, facing it in their own personal way (Messmer Uccelli, 2014).

From the perspective of developmental psychology, the diagnosis presents itself as a fracture not only in the identity of the individual, but also in the identity of the entire family system. Both the patient and his family find themselves having to redefine their identity, seeking a new balance in family relationships and facing the developmental tasks linked to the specific phase of the individual and family life cycle they are going through (de Ceuninck van Capelle et al., 2016; Kouzoupis et al., 2010; Rintell & Melito, 2013; Scabini et al., 2006).

As recently stated, it is only in recent times that some scientific studies have investigated the dynamics of changes in familial relationships in relation to MS. Particularly, in the first decade of the new millennium, some research was published that examined the effects of the disease on one's romantic partner, often examining situations of medium or severe disability and describing the difficulties experienced by the partner in the role of caregiver (Bogosian et al., 2009; Janssen et al., 2003; Liedström et al., 2010; Starks et al., 2010). Subsequently, studies moved to the topic of parenting, examining the effects of the parent's illness on their children (Bogosian et al., 2010; Boström & Nilsagård, 2016; Moberg et al., 2017; Pakenham & Cox, 2012); also in these studies, situations of medium-severe disability of the parent and the role of caregiver, in this case played by their child, were principally considered (Bjorgvinsdottir & Halldorsdottir, 2013). The effect of a child's illness on their parent remains minimally examined, and few existing works have been conducted on parents with pediatric children (Carroll et al., 2016; Hinton & Kirk, 2017; Messmer Uccelli et al., 2013). There are therefore no studies, other than ours which we will mention later (Calandri et al., 2022), that have focused on the psychological experiences of parents of young adult children with MS, despite the majority of diagnoses occurring between the ages of 20 and 30.

Therefore, in line with the growing attention to the psychological aspects of parenting in the presence of MS, our recent research and intervention interests have turned to the effects of the illness on the relationships between parents and children. Attention to this aspect, on which knowledge is scarce, was requested precisely by the intervention groups for the newly diagnosed: while some participants reported their experiences and difficulties as parents, others, as newly diagnosed young adults, reported their trying relationships with their own parents. Hence, we propose in this chapter the topic of parenting from two perspectives: one is that of the parent who has a young adult child with MS, and second that of the parent suffering from MS who must reconcile their parental role with the continuous challenges of their illness.

In the first part of the chapter, we will present a first exploratory thread of the project, started in 2017, intended for parents of young adult children with MS. In particular, we will illustrate the primary results from the interviews conducted, including the group intervention implemented with the parents starting from the themes that emerged from the interviews themselves.

In the second part of the chapter, we will describe a second exploratory thread of the project, started in 2019, aimed at parents with MS; we will illustrate some salient themes relating to being parents with this disease and we will describe the experience of the meetings specifically intended for them.

Being parents of a young adult child with MS (Federica Graziano)

As previously mentioned, the experience of parents with children diagnosed with MS has generally been little studied in the scientific literature. The few studies in this regard have dealt with parents with minor children diagnosed with MS (Carroll et al., 2016; Hinton & Kirk, 2017; Messmer Uccelli et al., 2013).

However, these studies are only partially helpful in understanding the experiences of parents who have a young adult child with MS. This is because the relationship between parents and young adult children is different than that of previous ages, and therefore demands specific attention. Young adults are at an age in which achieving independence from their family, not only from an economic point of view, but also emotionally and relationally, represents one of the principal objectives in one's development while one's illness poses a grand challenge in respect to this developmental process (Arnett, 2000). Usually, during young adulthood, parent–child relationships become increasingly equal, but a child's illness can lead the family system to intensify its dependence (Walsh, 1998, 2016), even more so in the Italian culture, characterized by a prolonged stay in the family of children often beyond the age of 30–35 (Crocetti & Meeus, 2014; EUROSTAT, 2019).

In the literature, there are studies that have analyzed the role of parent caregivers for their young adult children, but these concern chronic diseases or disabilities different than MS and the resulting indications cannot be applied tout court to this disease due to its elevated specificity. In particular, the very term "caregiver" is not fully suited to defining the role of parents to their young adult child with MS. These young people, in fact, usually do not have a physical disability that requires direct assistance, even if they report various psychological difficulties, which their parents inevitably have to contend with. Usually, parents of young adults with MS experience intense worries and uncertainties about the care their adult child may need in the near future. For this reason, some authors have spoken of the people close to young patients, including parents, as "anticipatory caregiver" (Strickland et al., 2015). The expression underscores how these individuals live a condition where they envision a change that may occur in their relationship with their ill family member, consequently anticipating a future representation of oneself as the caregiver. The identity of the family members therefore remains undefined precisely because it is linked to the uncertainty of the disease.

The relationship of parents with their young adult children affected by MS therefore presents specific characteristics that need to be explored in greater depth, to increase knowledge about the lives of people with this disease and to be able to plan support interventions aimed not only at young sufferers but also to their parents. Beginning with these considerations, we conducted semi-structured interviews with a sample of parents of newly diagnosed young adult patients to investigate in depth various aspects related to their experiences.

In the next three subparagraphs, we will expose these experiences, with particular reference to the three areas investigated by the interview: emotions and experiences at the time of diagnosis and in the current moment, quality of the relationship, representation of the future (see Box 5.1). Here, we will not go into detail about all the aspects that emerged from the analysis of the rich material of the interviews (for which we refer to the specific publications, see Calandri et al., 2022; Graziano et al., 2024), but the results that emerged will be highlighted in the three areas that seem most useful for application purposes, in particular for the implications they have for the planning and implementation of interventions to support parents.

The parents' experience at the time of diagnosis and now

One of the most difficult and delicate moments in the journey of a family facing MS is the diagnosis. The reaction of parents to the diagnosis of their child with MS seems to be very similar to the reaction reported by patients. Many parents report a sense of bewilderment and confusion or actual trauma ("It was a shock!"; "The world fell on me"; "I felt lost because I didn't know the disease"). This experience is often accompanied by an attitude of rejection, avoidance, and non-acceptance of the diagnosis ("We thought there was a mistake"; "I didn't think it was true, I didn't want to accept the situation"). The emotions most frequently reported by parents include fear – in all its shades: from worry, to anxiety, to feelings of actual panic

---

Box 5.1   Interviews with parents of newly diagnosed young adults: Participants and interview outline

Thirteen semi-structured interviews were conducted with parents of young adults with MS (eight mothers, five fathers, mean age 55, range 48–65), including four parental couples (the two parents were interviewed separately). Their children (nine in total) had a mean age of 24 (range 19–35) and were all living with their parents. From a clinical point of view, all children had a diagnosis of relapsing–remitting MS, with a mean duration of disease of 3.7 years and mild or moderate disability.

The interview investigated the following areas.

- The emotions and thoughts experienced by the parent when the child was diagnosed with MS and the emotions and thoughts experienced by the parent at the present time.
- The quality of the parent's relationship with the child, with particular attention to any difficulties and resources/strategies to manage these difficulties.
- The representation of the child's future and of one's own future as a parent.

The interviews lasted an average of one hour, were audio-recorded, transcribed in full and subjected to thematic analysis of the content (Braun & Clarke, 2006).

("A lot of worry about the unknown"; "A terrible fear") – and sadness – which sometimes takes the form of anguish and desperation ("I had a few moments of desperation"; "I spent several weeks crying"). In addition, a sense of guilt often appears, as emerges from the words of some fathers and mothers: the parent irrationally blames themself for what happened to their child, for having neglected the situation ("I experienced it with a sense of guilt because she had told us that she had vision problems, but at the beginning we didn't give it any weight") or for being somehow responsible for it ("Maybe I took some medicines during pregnancy that had this effect"). Many also report a sense of impotence, often linked to anxiety about the unknown that lies ahead ("You feel useless"; "It's like having a wall in front of you that you can't see beyond"). Finally, some parents report having felt a sense of liberation and relief at the diagnosis, especially when the path to the diagnosis was very long and tiring ("The diagnosis was a liberation for us") or when it allowed us to exclude fears of a diagnosis considered worse ("It was almost a relief"). It is interesting to emphasize how different experiences are sometimes present in the same person or follow one another over time, also in relation to the specific experience lived by the children and the individual characteristics of the individual parents.

At the time of the interview, several parents reported an experience oscillating between opposing emotions, often coexisting in the same individual, also with respect to the fluctuating course of their child's illness. Positive experiences include tranquility, acceptance and optimism, often associated with a stable state of the illness, the absence of relapses or the effectiveness of treatments ("I feel more relieved"; "I am calm and I trust in science"; "The experience of this moment is all in all quite serene"; "We see that our son is better and we are better too, perhaps we have even grown up together with the illness"). Negative experiences include worries and states of anxiety, linked above all to the uncertainty of the disease ("I am always afraid that he has new lesions"; "It is as if there is always a shadow"; "You are always stressed"), between a sense of impotence and a sensation of heaviness ("I am a little sad"; "I don't know what to say to my son"; "There is this weight, this burden that I wish was not there"). Finally, many parents report the concern of not letting their emotions show to their children, the need to appear calm and serene in their eyes, so as not to aggravate their emotional experience which is already often defeatist.

The relationship with a young adult child with MS: Between closeness and autonomy

Interviews with parents revealed the perception of illness as an additional challenge in the relationship with a young adult child. Parents must learn to relate to their child who is no longer an adolescent and who must find his or her own way, making autonomous choices in terms of study, work and emotional relationships. Illness intervenes complicating this path, which is already difficult for any young person, especially with regard to problems related to work and emotional relationships. Parents therefore find themselves in a challenging situation; they often report a sense of impotence and wonder about the best ways to help their children, both in matters more directly related to the illness and with respect to problems in everyday life.

The main difficulty expressed by most of the parents interviewed is to maintain a level of closeness to their child, appropriate to their age and illness, offering them emotional support but at the same time encouraging their autonomy, without being too detached or too intrusive. The delicate balance between recognizing the child's need for autonomy and yet care is perplexing to create and then maintain, while developing necessarily new adjustments.

From the analysis of the interviews, it emerges that some parents have an excessively protective attitude toward their child, not appropriate for his developmental stage. In particular, some parents seem to relate to their child as if he or she were still an adolescent or even a small child. In these cases, they themselves manage the therapies, take charge of solving any problems, making decisions on their behalf, often without engaging in a consultation with them.

At the beginning I called the department to make sure they didn't overlook the symptoms my son was reporting... (mother, 50 years old).

Since we didn't want him to climb stairs, we bought a stair lift to make it easier for him, but we didn't tell him and after trying it once, he never used it again (father, 59 years old).

The parent's overprotective attitude in some cases is accompanied by excessive control over their child, in relation to his/her stage of development, which does not respect their autonomy and in some cases becomes a real interference in the management of their daily life, not only related to the illness.

I go shopping for him, I buy him what he likes and I try to prepare a good lunch for him, so that he tries to eat healthily (mother, 54 years old).

In other cases, parents seem to show anticipatory anxiety regarding their child's health conditions, a concern that is excessive and more intense than that of the child themself.

With her illness I became much more apprehensive and stressed (mother, 48 years old).

In other cases, the parent is excessively indulgent and permissive toward the child, justifying their decisions and behaviors by attributing the reasons to their illness.

With the disease you give him a bit of everything, it's easier for him to get things (father, 59 years old).
I have always spoiled my daughter. If I can do something for her, if I can take a task off her shoulders, I do it! (mother, 48 years old).
Sometimes I realize that I justify her because of the illness (mother, 53 years old).

In some cases, the parent's overprotective attitude can lead to relational modalities in which a real symbiosis with the child emerges: the parent makes their child's experience and difficulties his/her own, replaces him/her in many daily activities and ends up living the illness as if it were his/her own. An example of this is this statement by a mother with a sick daughter:

I can't be detached in the relationship with her... it's as if I feel sick too (mother, 48 years old).

Other times, in interviews, some parents use the first person plural of the verb when talking about their child's illness experience, as in the example we report:

Now an important step that he must take... is that we must find a job (mother, 54 years old).

From the words of other parents, in contrast, emerges the ability to give support to their child, while at the same time encouraging their autonomy and respecting the boundaries of the relationship that is based on trust, mutual availability for dialogue and adequate emotional closeness.

The parent always feels like they have their child at home, but you have to realize that you have a 25-year-old man... (father, 56 years old).
A parent should have a supporting role, as a fighter alongside their child (mother, 53 years old).
I try to support her without being intrusive... I always try to do things a little on tiptoe, without being imposing (mother, 55 years old).

According to some parents interviewed, respect for their child's thoughts and opinions, for example regarding the illness and the therapies, is central to managing the relationship, even if it sometimes involves difficulties.

Now if he has relapses, I let him manage them as he wants... I try to respect his way of thinking (mother, 50 years old).

In particular, some parents perceive how difficult it is to balance closeness and autonomy when it comes to obtaining information from healthcare professionals about their child's illness, the evolution of the symptoms, the effectiveness of the treatments and their side effects. They feel the need to have information, but at the same time, they are aware that their desire risks coming into conflict with the protection of the privacy of their children, now adults, by health workers.

There are so many questions I have asked myself... about the symptoms, about the treatments... but obviously we are talking about a 28-year-old person so.... we need to.... adjust our aim... so as not to be intrusive, because she has her own life (mother, 55 years old).

Other parents justify their desire to have in-depth information from health workers with the need to be of help to their son.

If my son asks me questions about the treatments, I have to be ready... I would like to talk about it in private with the neurologist, because I have to be able to answer (father, 56 years old).

Parents often implement a slow process of change in their relationship with their children, in the direction of a progressively greater respect for their decision-making autonomy as adults.

Before, I actively tried to take care of him, I felt obliged to encourage him to do certain things... now I try to respect his choices (mother, 50 years old).

Dialogue with the child is the central tool for managing the relationship. The ability to express one's thoughts and moods with words and the willingness to listen to each other allow for better management of conflict between parents and children, conflict that the disease sometimes seems to have accentuated.

> *Now we are able to talk more, but on personal issues he withdraws into his shell... with the disease he has become much harder, more angular... (mother, 57 years old).*
>
> *He has always opposed any rule and from when he became ill, this attitude exploded (mother, 53 years old).*

On the contrary, some parents emphasize how, following the diagnosis, the relationship with their child has actually improved and has somehow strengthened.

> *At the beginning of the disease we were together a lot and this has brought us closer... now we tell each other everything (mother, 53 years old).*

Managing the relationship with a child suffering from MS can be facilitated when you can count on the support that comes from other family members and friends. On the contrary, when this social support is not present, the difficulties are greater.

> *After the diagnosis, the relationship with my husband was difficult... now it has improved, we can talk about our son's illness and we support each other (mother, 57 years old).*
>
> *In the family we are very close and we also have many friends so there is no risk of one being alone with their problems, but we can talk about them (mother, 55 years old).*
>
> *It is just me and my daughter, I have some friends, but it is never like having a family relationship, isolation is unfortunately a problem for both me and her (mother, 48 years old).*

The future of the child and the parents

Among the topics discussed with parents during the interviews, there is one that is particularly delicate in situations of chronic illness: the theme of the future. In fact, the representation that parents have about their children's future is profoundly influenced by the uncertainty and unpredictability of this illness. The dominant aspect that characterizes the representation of their children's future is ambivalence, which concerns both the course of the illness and the therapies and the planning of their working and emotional life. The fluctuating course of MS on the one hand seems to leave room, during periods of remission, for a life experience similar to that of other peers; on the other hand, uncertainty increases worries about the future which can lead to living in a situation of constant fear for possible relapses.

Some parents, for example, say:

> *You touch wood every time you have to go for tests, you have to do an MRI... and you hope that there isn't another lesion... (mother, 55 years old).*

But you know that there is this sword of Damocles that sooner or later will come and hit you on the head... so you always have this worry... (mother, 48 years old).

The invisible symptoms, first of all fatigue, are difficult to explain to other people, who may believe that the person is healthy, thus increasing the sense of isolation and alienation.

If you are not in a wheelchair then it is not multiple sclerosis, it is something else, you are fine ... the others do not understand (mother, 53 years old).

Even the therapies are subject to ambivalence because on the one hand, they allow to slow the progression of the disease but, on the other, they have side effects that are often more disabling than the symptoms themselves. For example, some say:

The therapy works very well ... clearly we are always a bit on edge because every six months he has to do these tests, always hoping that everything goes well ... (mother, 57 years old).
    In the event that this drug could no longer be used due to the risk of encephalitis, what would the side effects of a possible other therapy be? (father, 54 years old).

Therapies therefore represent both a resource and a constraint that limits the autonomy of young people, as is clear from this sentence:

The therapy, by forcing him to return once a month [to Italy], could cause problems in finding a job or taking courses abroad, since I don't know if this therapy could be done there (mother, 53 years old).

In particular, some parents fear that their son might interrupt the therapies to avoid side effects, as this mother reports:

I hope that he continues to be treated... because sometimes they get lost during the treatments... I hope that he continues to be treated, that his life continues like this, that's it... (mother, 57 years old).

With regard to autonomy and independence, some parents may oscillate between the idea of their child with all the potential and possibilities of a person with a chronic disease that is not particularly disabling, and the idea of a future characterized by serious physical disability:

It is true that I keep an eye on the fact of being able to have some money aside to build an elevator in the house, to be able to have some money aside to equip the ground floor for him and... I like that, how can I say, from a practical point of view, I have these thoughts but he... he lives normally, so much so that he came to the city to live alone so... I mean, what can I say? It's fine like this... (mother, 53 years old).

Ambivalence also characterizes the representation of a child's future in the workplace. Sometimes, the young adult children of our interviewees are engaged in work activities and the parents do not know how to advise them about when and how to inform the employer or colleagues about their illness: doing this could expose them to a risk of discrimination or stigmatization. But, on the other hand, it could allow them to take advantage of the benefits, in terms of working conditions and permits, useful for the management of their illness itself. The following sentences exemplify these aspects well.

To the normal worry that all of us parents have about our son being unemployed for a long time, we add the problem of illness (father, 56 years old).
The problem is that once he graduates, if he has to go to a job interview, should he say so? Shouldn't he say so? Is it better he sign up for special job placement lists or not? That is, face the reality of life in this sense. (mother, 57 years old).

Finally, ambivalence also characterizes expectations regarding affective relationships. Parents recognize that the presence of a partner could have a supportive function for their children, but they are also concerned that their children may meet a person who is unable to understand the difficulties of living with MS. Some parents say:

I hope he finds a girl who understands his situation (father, 59 years old).
I am worried... that [she] will be disabled, that she will not have a family (mother, 48 years old).

Even projects related to parenthood, in particular the choice to undertake a pregnancy, are characterized by strong ambivalence: some parents, on the one hand, would be ready to support their daughters who decide to become mothers, even if, on the other, they have strong fears about the difficulties that would inevitably be added to those of the disease. For example, a mother says:

I hope she has a family, I hope she has someone to share her life with, I hope she has children, even if I think they are too tiring... I don't know... when she tells me: «I would like to have children», I think to myself: «Please don't let her have any, no, no children!» but I tell her: «You do it!», I support her... (mother, 48 years old).

The theme of the future does not only concern the growth prospects of children with MS, but also concerns the life projects that parents themselves develop for themselves. This representation is usually deeply influenced by the child's illness and its uncertainty. As we have already said, parents of young adults with MS often have children who present few or no disabling symptoms, but they know that the illness may worsen over time. For this reason, they often imagine having to provide care to their child especially in the future, but the uncertainty of the illness does not allow them to establish if and when this will be necessary. From the analysis of the themes that emerged from the interviews with parents, we can describe three main representations of their future:

1   Absence of future planning.
2   Presence of planning, but strongly conditioned by the child's illness.
3   Presence of planning despite the child's illness.

As for the lack of planning, some parents say they do not think about their future, because they are too worried about the present. These parents seem to live in a state of a developmental block, which does not allow them to think of themselves as individuals changing toward significant goals; consequently, they cannot imagine any future plan. Some parents confirm:

I have no plans because... I don't know... I live day by day (father, 65 years old).
  I never make plans because... then maybe the plans fall... like papers falling down... I mean, I'd like to make plans, but I'm always afraid I won't be able to make them happen... (father, 49 years old).

Other parents, on the other hand, think about their future, but their plans are all strongly centered on their child's illness and its possible evolution: some think of reducing their commitments at work, others of saving money and modifying their home to eliminate architectural barriers in view of a worsening of their child's disabilities. The future is essentially seen as the time to manage a more serious illness than how it manifests itself in the present.

For my future everything is tied to my son (mother, 57 years old).
  The company I work for offered me a job abroad, but I have to realize that with a family situation like this, with my son who may need assistance ok, it's not like I can pretend he's not there... what would happen if my son had a serious relapse while I'm abroad? (father, 56 years old).
  I make sure I have some money put aside to build an elevator in the house, to equip the ground floor for him... I have these thoughts from a practical point of view. (mother, 53 years old).

Finally, there are also parents who have a representation of their future that is not centered only on their child's illness. They try to preserve a personal plan, without denying the presence of the illness: it represents a challenge for their future, but also an opportunity to improve family relationships and find positive aspects in their lives. In these interviews, the need for parents to safeguard personal living spaces to be cultivated also for the greater well-being of the family itself emerges.

> *I see in my future that every now and then my husband and I... we leave, we go away, for two days, three days, because old age will be made up of me and my husband, we hope, and if we are well we will be able to be of help to our son (mother, 54 years old).*
>
> *At this moment I would have this course abroad and I would feel like doing it, even with my sick daughter, in the sense that now I see that she is well and therefore I would feel like doing it... this is a dream that I would have... I repeat... I do not experience my daughter's situation as something to give up, absolutely not (mother, 53 years old).*

From research to intervention: Guidelines for supporting parents of young adult patients

The rich textual material collected through the interviews allowed us to identify the main critical issues experienced by parents with a young adult child with MS and to develop indications for a psychological support intervention to be implemented in a group. At a general level, it is important that, together with the care of young adult patients, the possibility of a support path is also offered to their parents. This global care of the patient and the people close to him can help all members of the family system to face the challenge posed by the diagnosis of MS.

First of all, parents, like patients, need to have information about MS and therapies to help them understand their child's illness; this knowledge allows them to strengthen their sense of self-efficacy and control of the situation given the illness that involves them as parents. An intervention specifically dedicated to parents allows them to ask questions and discuss with a professional and with each other, without their children present, and therefore feel free and less apprehensive toward violating their children's privacy. This discussion can subsequently open up spaces for discussion with their children, where parents feel they can manage their role more effectively.

As we have addressed, the parents interviewed experienced several negative emotions at the time of their children's diagnosis; even the experiences reported at the time of the interview are characterized by contrasting emotions, often difficult to manage. From a perspective of supporting families with young adult children with MS, the issue of managing emotions is therefore of central importance and it is necessary to think about interventions to strengthen this ability. Parents who are better equipped to manage emotions will be able to regulate the relationship with their child more effectively, especially with regard to the difficult dynamic balance between closeness and emotional support on the one hand and the promotion of autonomy on the other.

Connected to this aspect, another particularly critical dimension for parents emerged from the analysis of the interviews: their ability to communicate effectively with their children, not only regarding the disease. Support interventions should therefore also aim to increase parents' ability to communicate effectively, which, in turn, would promote a supportive dynamic in the parent–child relationship.

Within this supportive relationship, the parent should be ready to support the child in their future choices, trying to take their point of view, but not replacing them. Furthermore, it is important that parents do not identify themselves exclusively in the role of caregiver, a situation in which they often adopt negative and catastrophic thoughts about their child's future, and by extension about their own future, but rather preserve their individual and couple planning, "despite" their child's illness. Parents should also therefore be supported in a process of redefining their personal and parental identity, in the search for goals that can give meaning to their life.

Group intervention for parents of young adults with MS (Martina Borghi)

Starting from the reflections that emerged from the interviews, we designed and implemented a pilot program for parents with a young adult child suffering from MS. The main objective was to provide a space for discussion between parents with the guidance of a psychologist and to provide some tools to help parents manage the relationship with their child. The intervention was based on the same theoretical approach that guides the intervention with patients: the disease as a challenge in the evolutionary cycle of the individual and the family, the individual as protagonist in their own development. The intervention had the goal of helping parents in the process of adapting to the disease, a process that concerns not only the child, but also themselves. Adapting to their child's MS also implies that parents redefine their own identity, not focusing only on the disease, and find appropriate ways to understand their child in relation to the challenges their illness presents. Parents are therefore also required to learn to live with the illness, while keeping their experience separate from that of their child.

The intervention was structured in four group meetings (6–10 participants), which took place every two weeks. The meetings were conducted by a psychologist following an open and flexible path that was adopted during the group discussions in relation to the themes that emerged. An observer was present at the meetings who took note of the contents covered and the group dynamics; for this purpose, the observer filled out a specific observation sheet, structured in a similar way to that used in the groups for newly diagnosed people.

Specifically, the intervention had the following objectives:

- provide parents with some information about the disease and therapies;
- encourage reflection on the characteristics of the relationship with a young adult child and the difficulties posed by their illness and
- enhance parental self-efficacy in the relationship with a young adult child with this illness.

All the meetings opened and closed with relaxation and breathing exercises to mark the beginning and end of a specially dedicated time, in which people mentally prepare to enter and participate, and from which permits them to return to everyday life.

During the meetings, various topics were addressed, always according to a comparison method of the facilitator with the participants and of the participants among themselves. The topics were proposed in a flexible way also in relation to the requests that emerged from the group.

First, basic information was provided regarding the characteristics of the disease and the therapies. For some specific topics on which questions were asked (for example, disability practices, the regulations for renewing the driving license), directions were given to find clear and correct information via the Internet.

In addition to this information, much space has been dedicated to the psychological difficulties generally encountered by young patients: for example, the worries and anxieties, the difficulty in talking about it with parents, the risk of denial of the illness, the possible presence of angry attitudes toward the parent, excessive self-limitation or, on the contrary, defiance, provoking attitudes. Parents had the opportunity to reflect on their specific life situations, finding themselves in the points touched upon. The focus of the reflection was the meaning of the illness in relation to the moment of personal development that young adults are going through, characterized by the need to gain increasing autonomy and redefine their identity in the transition to full adulthood.

Starting from these considerations, we talked about the parents' experiences and their relationship with their children. Parents generally feel anxious, sometimes they feel guilty, they are worried about their child's future. The difficulty often expressed by parents is that of maintaining an adequate closeness to their child, so as to be able to be supportive without being excessively protective. The main objective was therefore to help parents better understand some of their experiences, trying to separate them from those of their children, with the ultimate goal of being helpful to them and promoting their autonomy. During the meetings, some tools were provided to allow parents to feel more competent in their relationship with their child. Often, materials similar to those used with patients were proposed, adapted in form and content to the specific situation of the parents. In other cases, we developed specific materials, also created by starting from the findings that emerged in the parent interviews. In the following subparagraphs, we report some examples.

Learning to recognize your emotions in critical situations

Examples of critical situations involving the child were given (for example, the onset of a new attack, suddenly not feeling well without an understanding of the cause, the child's decision to do something the parent does not approve of). Parents were asked to express their experience in each situation, trying to distinguish between physical sensation, emotion, thought and behavior. Parents were then asked, if they wished, to present other significant situations in their experience, trying to reflect on their usual ways of an emotional reaction and how directly these reactions can affect one's well-being or discomfort.

How to behave in situations with strong emotional resonance

Starting from these concrete situations, some reflections were shared with parents on the most appropriate ways to manage emotions that are a source of suffering and how to promote positive ones. The usefulness of avoiding activating habitual response patterns that may be dysfunctional, is to take a breath to better focus on the problem, to consider possible solutions, to choose the most suitable and viable solution, evaluating its usefulness over time.

Some critical situations in the relationship with children

Beginning with some ideas that emerged from the interviews, we presented parents with some examples of critical situations that can arise in the relationship alongside a young adult child with MS (for example, a job offer far from home, the choice to spend a period of study abroad, the choice to communicate the diagnosis to their employer). Then, parents were invited to reflect on their possible reactions if they found themselves in a similar situation and what may be possible positive and negative consequences of such reactions.

To help your child with programming

A small guide was proposed to parents to help their child and support them in their planning in the different areas of life, with the final goal of promoting their autonomy, taking into account the constraints of the illness. We reflected with the parents on the need to help their child find specific goals that can be important and significant for them, but at the same time achievable, making an effort to see reality from their point of view and not from their own. We also discussed the importance of identifying with their child effective strategies and aids that can allow these goals to be achieved. The key assumption, for parents, should be to give help to the child only if they request it, or is open to receiving it, not to supersede them in solving problems or planning activities.

To promote good communication between parents and children

With the parents, we reflected on the need to have clear and effective communication with their children, in which meanings are shared, avoiding the risks of ambiguity and misunderstandings. Also in this case, both imaginary situations were proposed, and personal situations were asked to be presented, if the participants wanted to share them with the group. In keeping with the theme of communication, we also worked, as previously, on the need to not confuse one's own objectives with those of their child, always with a view to differentiation from the child, consideration of their point of view and respect for their sphere of intimacy.

The evaluation of this first pilot program was based on what emerged from the participants in the final meeting including the internal comparison within our working group. The experience can be considered positive from several points of view: parents in general evaluated the meetings as an opportunity for comparison, in which it was possible to share doubts and moods with the other participants, feeling at ease, without needing to hide their experiences, as sometimes happens in the relationship with their child or with other family members. The support and guidance of the psychologist were critically useful for deepening some experiences and for finding more appropriate strategies pertinent to managing tensions in their relationship with children. The most evident criticality encountered both by our working group and by some participants was the difficulty in creating a more dynamic group dimension, due to the heterogeneity of the family histories of the participants. In some cases, the comparison between parents was reserved consequently, the discussion sometimes remained on a general level. Understandably, going into more detail would have meant bringing into play specific aspects of one's family history.

The overall experience has confirmed how important it is to work with parents of young adult patients to contend with their illness within a comprehensive care of the patient and of the systems of relationships in which they are inserted. Taking full charge allows for positive repercussions to be triggered both on the patient and on their family members, who often feel excluded and at the same time do not know how to help without being intrusive in their child's life. The group dimension seems to be useful to facilitate sharing and discussion, although in order to benefit from it to the fullest it is necessary to try to form groups that are as homogeneous as possible (for example, based on the age of the children or the duration of their illness). Finally, planning maintenance meetings over time would give continuity to the experience, providing the opportunity for parents to meet up again, to share the changes that have occurred and to continue the discussion guided by the psychologist.

Parenthood with MS (Emanuela Calandri)

In the previous paragraphs, we have discussed the topic of parenthood considering the parents of young adults with MS. However, there is also another reality in which parenthood is linked to the disease: when the parent is ill. In this second situation, we may find ourselves faced with two further conditions: parents who receive the diagnosis having already had children, or people who choose to become parents at a later time after diagnosis. In this part of the chapter, we will delve into these two specific life experiences.

MS and the parental role: Difficulties and resources

Only in recent years have some studies examined the parental function in people suffering from MS; in particular, the experience of mothers who have children of different ages, born before the diagnosis of the disease. At present, the experience of fathers with MS remains largely unexplored, firstly because MS affects women more and studies are conducted on predominantly female samples; furthermore, childcare duties continue to be largely borne by women, especially when the children are small. All this does not exclude that the scope of studies should broaden and examine the management of the paternal role with the disease (Bove et al., 2016).

From the studies in the literature, as well as from our work, it emerges that being a parent with MS implies additional difficulties to the demanding educational task of mothers and fathers. The different symptoms of MS, first of all fatigue and motor problems, relapses and constant worries about the unpredictable course of the disease, represent an additional burden compared to the performance of the parental role, regardless of the age of the children. If on the one hand fatigue affects above all the activities of caring for young children, shared play and the ability to accompany children to school or to leisure activities (Pakenham et al., 2012), on the other hand the presence of the illness and the worries associated with it affect the relationship with children even when they are older.

In particular, parents may experience feelings of guilt and inadequacy because they perceive that they are no longer able to take care of their children as they did before the illness. In a study examining the impact of fatigue on the performance of parenting tasks (Haynes-Lawrence & West, 2018), mothers and fathers report being frustrated primarily because fatigue prevents them from engaging in activities with their children as they would like and as they did when they were not ill. Furthermore, fatigue also has a negative impact on the educational strategies implemented with their children; as a result, parents feel less effective in carrying out their educational role compared to the period before their diagnosis. For example, many report having allowed their children to use technological devices excessively for entertainment, which in turn causes frustration and increased guilt (Haynes-Lawrence & West, 2018). For some parents, guilt is also accompanied by an experience of loss, caused by not being able to fully participate in family activities and having to delegate a series of additional responsibilities and commitments to the other parent (Pakenham & Cox, 2012). The sense of inadequacy, which can be present in all parents in certain circumstances, appears in a more accentuated form in parents with MS, so much so that they develop the doubt of not being "good parents".

Parents with MS, therefore, experience concerns not only about their own health, but also about how the disease affects their ability to dedicate themselves to their children, and these concerns can increase depressive symptoms (Harrison & Stuifbergen, 2002). In this regard, the results of our in-depth research, presented in Chapter 4, also highlighted how mothers participating in the study reported greater depressive symptoms and lower well-being than women without children. The double burden of the disease and the parental role can therefore have negative repercussions on adaptation to the disease, especially when it is not adequately taken into consideration by the patients themselves and especially by those who must take care of them (Haynes-Lawrence & West, 2018; Payne & McPherson, 2010).

Parents with MS therefore face the "double challenge" of coping with the disease and at the same time carrying out their educational role. In this complex dual challenge, the ability of parents to redefine their identity as parents with a chronic disease plays a central role, with the recognition of the limits and possibilities that this condition entails. The central role of identity in adapting to the disease in mothers is a result that emerged from one of our research studies presented in Chapter 4. In fact, we observed how greater satisfaction with one's identity is linked to fewer depressive feelings and greater well-being especially for women with children. The central role of redefining identity for mothers with MS was also highlighted in a study on the links between MS and being a mother (Willson et al., 2018). Mothers who are able to redefine their identity in relation to the limits of the disease experience a lower sense of inadequacy in the relationship with their children. Furthermore, they perceive themselves as different or inferior in comparison with other mothers less frequently, and this reduces the fear of social stigma, positively influencing their adaptation to the disease.

Studies on parenting in MS also highlight another very important aspect: the role of social support. It constitutes one of the main resources for dealing with the difficulties of being a parent with MS (Pakenham et al., 2012). In fact, in addition to the relief in care practices, the parent's worries and sense of inadequacy are reduced when he or she can count on the practical and emotional support of their partner, extended family or other significant others (Harrison & Stuifbergen, 2002; Kosmala-Anderson & Wallace, 2013). This leads us to reflect on the importance of the family and social network for the parent with MS, an aspect that should not be overlooked when taking care of a patient affected by this chronic disease.

Choosing motherhood with MS

As we saw in Chapter 4, the interest of psychological literature in the topic of being mothers with MS is relatively recent, even though the disease is diagnosed mainly in women in a phase of the life cycle in which many are considering the possibility of motherhood. While until a few years ago pregnancy was considered precluded to women with MS, the progress of medical knowledge has changed this opinion and psychological studies have also begun to be interested in the topic of the choice of motherhood for women affected by this chronic disease (Amato et al., 2017; Ghezelhesari et al., 2024; Özkan & Polat Dünya, 2023; Payne & McPherson, 2010; Prunty et al., 2008).

Scientific studies in recent decades have provided answers to the main questions that women with MS ask themselves in relation to a possible pregnancy. First of all, the questions concern the possible effect of MS on fertility, on the course of pregnancy and on childbirth, as well as the presence of any risks for the child. Evidence in the literature highlights how MS does not compromise fertility, even if therapies can have an influence on it. Furthermore, having MS does not in itself imply a greater probability of having a risky pregnancy: no greater risks of miscarriage, fetal death, neonatal mortality or fetal complications have been observed. Finally, the risk that a child with a parent with MS may in turn develop the disease is slightly higher than for those with a healthy parent, but it is a risk that does not exceed 5% (Canibaño et al., 2020).

Other questions from future mothers concern the effect of pregnancy on the disease, in particular whether pregnancy can modify the course of the disease and affect the occurrence of relapses, the appearance of new lesions and the severity of disability. On these points too, the evidence in the literature highlights how pregnancy does not alter the long-term course of the disease; in particular, an increase in disability linked to pregnancy has not been demonstrated. During pregnancy, women generally have fewer relapses. However, some typical symptoms, such as fatigue, difficulty walking and bladder and intestinal problems can worsen. There is a risk of relapse in the first six months after giving birth, presumably in relation to hormonal changes that influence the immune system (Canibaño et al., 2020; Langer-Gould, 2019; Schubert et al., 2023).

All studies in this regard highlight the importance for women to receive correct and adequate information.

Despite these reassurances about the course of pregnancy, very similar to physiological pregnancies, women with MS often experience the desire for motherhood and pregnancy with strong ambivalence: on the one hand, the joy of the possibility of becoming mothers, but on the other, strong fears for their own health and that of the child. Added to these concerns is also that related to the social judgment of others, especially family and friends (Carvalho et al., 2014; Kosmala-Anderson & Wallace, 2013). This aspect is particularly important because the choice of pregnancy, when you have MS, does not only concern the couple, but necessarily also involves the network of people you will need after giving birth (Lavorgna et al., 2020). Fears related to the management of the newborn also have a strong impact on the choice to undertake a pregnancy despite the disease; these women often fear that they cannot be "good mothers" due to the limits imposed by MS (Willson et al., 2018).

The postpartum period, very demanding for all mothers, risks being more tiring for women with MS. It is therefore essential for future mothers to prepare for this phase, trying to have the resources and social support necessary to take care of the baby, as well as themselves.

Pregnancy with MS can therefore be accompanied by physical and emotional difficulties, but the disease itself does not represent an obstacle to the decision to have children. Having adequate information and psychological support, both from significant people and from professionals, is a fundamental aspect in facing a choice, such as motherhood, which commits the person for their whole existence, since one is a parent forever.

Communicating the illness to one's children

The topic of communication is a fundamental component when talking about adaptation to chronic disease. One of the central dilemmas experienced by people with MS is whether to "tell" or not to tell family members, relatives, friends or work colleagues about the disease. When one decides to disclose one's condition, doubts arise about how much to explain about the disease and the best ways to communicate certain aspects, depending on the interlocutor and the relational context (for example, family of origin, partner, employer, colleagues, health workers). A further critical issue is represented by the ways in which to ask for help, an action that makes it possible to benefit from a social support network, and therefore achieve a better adaptation to the disease. These aspects were addressed in Chapter 2, and we have seen how they occupy a large space in our proposal for group intervention.

When people with MS also have a parental role, the issue of communicating the disease becomes particularly complicated. One of the major concerns for parents with MS, in fact, is linked to the choice of when to communicate their illness to children, as well as what to say and through what methods.

It often happens that parents decide to "say nothing", especially when the symptoms are not visible and it is thought that the children would not be able to understand, especially if they are still young. This choice is generally justified by the desire to protect the children from the pain of learning about the parent's illness; in reality, it is above all a self-defense, felt as necessary in the face of the difficulty of speaking openly about a personal condition not yet accepted and integrated into one's existence. However, hiding or denying this knowledge has negative consequences in both the short and long terms. In fact, children, even if at an early age, are able to perceive the changes that occur in their main context of life, which is the family, they perceive the parent's state of mind, or they realize that the parent "is no longer the same as before". The parent, for example, due to fatigue, no longer dedicates themselves to shared activities as they did before, and this can be interpreted by the child as laziness or, in more extreme cases, as a lack of attention and affection. Even young children notice that something has changed, for example in family habits and routines. Or, children, especially older ones, see that their parent takes drugs, sometimes through injections, or that they go to the hospital every now and then, and this can cause them to be very worried, which can lead them to believe that their parent is even about to die. With adolescent children, one can fall into the error of taking some information about the illness for granted, but even if their child does not ask questions or does not express their concerns openly, this does not mean that they do not have concerns about the parent's health. The parent's "not saying" can contribute to greatly increasing the children's worries, or to making them give themselves incorrect explanations that are sometimes worse than reality, or to blaming themselves for what is happening (Paliokosta et al., 2009).

Children must be recognized as having the right to know and understand what is happening in the family; to this end, it is essential that sincere, clear communication is established between parents and children, appropriate to the age of the children themselves, their level of maturity and their ability to understand. Children must be allowed to ask questions to better understand what is happening; the answers will be more effective the simpler, more essential and more useful they are for the current moment that the children are experiencing (Nilsagård & Boström, 2015).

For example, with younger children, talking about MS in scientific terms is not very effective. Instead, you can explain the most obvious symptoms and what happens when mom or dad is not feeling well. It can also be useful to read a fairy tale or look at an illustrated book together (there are materials designed specifically for this purpose, but all those fairy tales in which a situation of illness emerges can be good): the story allows you to start talking about it indirectly and in a way that is appropriate for the child's cognitive and emotional developments. As the child grows older, other tools can be used (for example, brochures, videos, documentaries) that can help the parent talk to the child about MS, in a way that is appropriate for his or her age and ability to understand. With adolescents, it is necessary to give more detailed information, because information that is too vague could increase their anxiety about the parent's health. For example, if necessary, the children could feel reassured by knowing the function of the medicine that the parent is taking. It is necessary for the parent to communicate to the child what the child really wants to know, without creating further disorientation (Bogosian et al., 2011; Mauseth & Hjälmhult, 2016; Razaz et al., 2014).

Through communication about a parent's illness, children are able to give meaning and significance to what is happening to them. Communicating with children about the illness is not a one-time event, but an ongoing process. Over time, children and teenagers will ask new questions and have new concerns; it is the parents' job to keep communication open and provide their children with the answers they ask for, possibly also resorting to the help of professionals if they find themselves in difficulty. Laying the foundations of dialogue on these topics when children are young can help to continue along a path that will certainly not be free of difficulties and obstacles.

Children, especially as they grow older, may take on a protective attitude toward the ill parent and not ask questions or express their concerns so as not to further burden the parent. It may also happen that they take on more responsibilities than required for their age and therefore constant attention must be paid to their emotional experience. Children of ill parents often develop a greater sense of responsibility and demonstrate greater empathy than their peers who do not experience a situation of illness in the family (Pakenham & Cox, 2012). These are positive aspects that however must always be proportional to the age of the children and young people, avoiding the generation of feelings of guilt or the limitation of the children's need to gradually gain autonomy from their parents (Moberg et al., 2017).

In communicating between parent and child regarding the illness, it is particularly useful to maintain a positive attitude that does not only underline what the illness takes away, but also and above all what can continue to be done in the family "despite the illness". In this situation, the parent with MS, supported by other members of the family system, has the opportunity to teach their children strategies to deal with difficulties, maintaining a positive attitude (Bonino, 2021).

Support meetings for parents with MS (Martina Borghi)

In light of what has been reported so far, it is really important to provide psychological support interventions for parents with MS, both for parenting planning and for managing the parental function. Our working group focused on the latter aspect, organizing, as a pilot experience, some meetings aimed at parents with MS with the aim of strengthening their self-efficacy in dealing with the difficulties experienced in the role of parent with the disease.

In this section, we will describe the experience of these meetings intended for patients with children under the age of 13, regardless of whether they were born before or after the diagnosis, and open to their respective partners, with a view to shared management, at the couple level, of the difficulties of the disease and parental tasks. The meetings were led by a psychologist, who followed an open path adaptable to the themes that would emerge in the group and to the life stories of the participants. The presence of an observer was foreseen who took note of the contents that emerged and the group dynamics, according to a path similar to that used in the meetings with the patients.

The meetings, of which there were two, were attended by both mothers and fathers affected by MS and also some partners; all had children between the ages of one and seven.

In the first meeting, after the introductions and the explanation of the group's objectives, participants were asked to share their story of the decision to become parents, bringing out personal experiences, doubts and uncertainties, but also the positive aspects. Different stories emerged, as expected, between mothers and fathers, but also between those who had children after the diagnosis, and those who were already parents at the time of the diagnosis. From the words of the participants, it emerged that the decision to become a mother – and to a lesser extent that of a father – had been closely linked to the support perceived and received from their family members and from healthcare personnel, in particular from the neurologist and the gynecologist. The mothers generally spoke positively about the experience of pregnancy, without denying the difficulties. For all of them, it was a matter of realizing their own life project, strongly desired, despite the illness.

Then, the group discussion moved on to the current experience of parents, in particular the difficulties in reconciling parental duties with the need to have space for oneself to cope with the difficulties of the disease. These difficulties are reported by both mothers and fathers, especially when there are very young children or more than one child. A central topic was the importance of family support (from the partner and the extended family), essential for managing the burden of parental duties and that of the illness.

The second and final meeting focused on the topic of communicating the disease to children, asking participants to share their experiences in this regard: they were then asked if they had spoken to their children about the disease, what they had said and in what ways. Some had spoken to their children about the disease, in a way that was appropriate for their age, others had only given explanations about the drugs. Some parents used videos, documentaries or books, in relation to the age, characteristics and interests of their children, finding in these tools a help in communicating with them. In some cases, the negative effect of not speaking to children about the parent's disease emerged. Sometimes, the importance of communicating with teachers and other family members also emerged, in order to create educational alliances between significant people in their children's lives.

The group, which was immediately very close-knit, allowed for a useful comparison between the participants and proved to be a source of help for the members in greater difficulty. This pilot experience confirmed the importance of this type of meeting and the need to continue in this direction.

References

Amato, M. P., Bertolotto, A., Brunelli, R., Cavalla, P., Goretti, B., Marrosu, M. G., Patti, F., Pozzilli, C., Provinciali, L., Rizzo, N., Strobelt, N., Tedeschi, G., Trojano, M., & Comi, G. (2017). Management of pregnancy-related issues in multiple sclerosis patients: The need for an interdisciplinary approach. *Neurological Sciences, 38*, 1849–1858.

Arnett, J. J. (2000). Emerging adulthood: A theory of development from the late teens through the twenties. *American Psychologist, 55*, 469–480.

Bjorgvinsdottir, K., & Halldorsdottir, S. (2013). Silent, invisible and unacknowledged: Experiences of young caregivers of single parents diagnosed with multiple sclerosis. *Scandinavian Journal of Caring Sciences, 28*(1), 38–48.

Bogosian, A., Moss-Morris, R., Bishop, F. L., & Hadwin, J. (2011). How do adolescents adjust to their parent's multiple sclerosis? An interview study. *British Journal of Health Psychology, 16*, 430–444.

Bogosian, A., Moss-Morris, R., & Hadwin, J. (2010). Psychosocial adjustment in children and adolescents with a parent with multiple sclerosis: A systematic review. *Clinical Rehabilitation, 24*, 789–801.

Bogosian, A., Moss-Morris, R., Yardley, L., & Dennison, L. (2009). Experiences of partners of people in the early stages of multiple sclerosis. *Multiple Sclerosis, 15*, 876–884.

Bonino, S. (2021). *Coping with chronic illness. Theories, issues and lived experiences.* Routledge.

Boström, K., & Nilsagård, Y. (2016). A family matter - when a parent is diagnosed with multiple sclerosis. A qualitative study. *Journal of Clinical Nursing, 25*, 1053–1061.

Bove, R., McHenry, A., Hellwig, K., Houtchens, M., Razaz, N., Smyth, P., Tremlett, H., Sadovnick, A. D., & Rintell, D. (2016). Multiple sclerosis in men: Management considerations. *Journal of Neurology, 263*, 263–273.

Braun, V., & Clarke, V. (2006). Using thematic analysis in psychology. *Qualitative Research in Psychology, 3*, 77–101.

Calandri, E., Graziano, F., Borghi, M., & Bonino, S. (2022). The future between difficulties and resources. Exploring parents' perspective on young adults with multiple sclerosis. *Family Relations, 71*(2), 686–706.

Canibaño, B., Deleu, D., Mesraoua, B., Melikyan, G., Ibrahim, F., & Hanssens, Y. (2020). Pregnancy-related issues in women with multiple sclerosis: An evidence-based review with practical recommendations. *Journal of Drug Assessment, 23*, 20–36.

Carroll, S., Chalder, T., Hemingway, C., Heyman, I., & Moss-Morris, R. (2016). "It feels like wearing a giant sandbag." Adolescent and parent perceptions of fatigue in paediatric multiple sclerosis. *European Journal of Paediatric Neurology, 20*, 938–945.

Carvalho, A. T., Veiga, A., Morgado, J., Tojal, R., Rocha, S., Vale, J., Sá, M. J., & Timóteo, A. (2014). Multiple sclerosis And motherhood choice: An observational study in Portuguese women patients. *Revista de Neurologia, 59*, 537–42.

Crocetti, E., & Meeus, W. (2014). "Family Comes First!" Relationships with family and friends in Italian emerging adults. *Journal of Adolescence, 37*, 463–1473.

de Ceuninck van Capelle, A., Visser, L. H., & Vosman, F. (2016). Multiple sclerosis (MS) in the life cycle of the family: An interpretative phenomenological analysis of the perspective of persons with recently diagnosed MS. *Families, Systems and Health, 34*(4), 435–440.

EUROSTAT (2019). *When are they ready lo leave the nest?* European Commission. https://ec.europa.eu/eurostat/web/products-eurostat-news/-/EDN-20190514-1

Ghezelhesari, E. M., Heydari, A., Ebrahimipour, H., Nahayati, M. A., & Khadivzadeh, T. (2024). Meta-synthesis of the motherhood-related needs of women with multiple sclerosis. *BMC Women's Health, 24*(1), 559.

Graziano, F., Borghi, M., Bonino, S., & Calandri, E. (2024). Parenting emerging adults with multiple sclerosis: A qualitative analysis of the Parents' perspective. *Journal of Child and Family Studies, 33*, 2367–2382.

Harrison, T., & Stuifbergen, A. (2002). Disability, social support, and concern for children: Depression in mothers with multiple sclerosis. *Journal of Obstetric, Gynecologic and Neonatal Nursing*, *31*, 444–453.

Haynes-Lawrence, D., & West, A. (2018). Managing fatigue in parents with multiple sclerosis. *Journal of Child and Family Studies*, 27, 1640–1649.

Hinton, D., & Kirk, S. (2017). Living with uncertainty and hope: A qualitative study exploring parents' experiences of living with childhood multiple sclerosis. *Chronic Illness*, *13*, 88–99.

Janssen, A. C. J. W., van Doorn, P. A., de Boer, J. B., van der Meche, F. G. A., Passchier, J., & Hintzen, R. Q. (2003). Impact of recently diagnosed multiple sclerosis on quality of life, anxiety, depression, and distress of patients and partners. *Acta Neurologica Scandinavica*, *108*, 389–395.

Kosmala-Anderson, J., & Wallace, L. M. (2013). A qualitative study of the childbearing experience of women living with multiple sclerosis. *Disability and Rehabilitation*, *35*, 976–981.

Kouzoupis, A. B., Paparrigopoulos, T., Soldatos, M., & Papadimitriou, G. N. (2010). The family of the multiple sclerosis patient: A psychosocial perspective. *International Review of Psychiatry*, *22*, 83–89.

Langer-Gould, A. M. (2019). Pregnancy and family planning in multiple sclerosis. *Continuum*, *25*, 773–792.

Lavorgna, L., Morra, V. B., & Margherita, G. (2020). Multiple sclerosis and maternity: A psychological explorative qualitative research. *The Qualitative Report*, *24*(5), 1279–1293.

Liedström, E., Isaksson, A. K., & Ahlström, G. (2010). Quality of life in spite of an unpredictable future: The next of kin of patients with multiple sclerosis. *Journal of Neuroscience Nursing*, *42*, 331–41.

Mauseth, T., & Hjälmhult, E. (2016). Adolescents' experiences on coping with parental multiple sclerosis: A grounded theory study. *Journal of Clinical Nursing*, *25*, 856–65.

Messmer Uccelli, M. (2014). The impact of multiple sclerosis on family members: A review of the literature. *Neurodegenerative Disease Management*, *4*, 177–185.

Messmer Uccelli, M., Traversa, S., Trojano, M., Viterbo, R. G., Ghezzi, A., & Signori, A. (2013). Lack of information about multiple sclerosis in children can impact parents' sense of competency and satisfaction within the couple. *Journal of the Neurological Sciences*, *15*, 100–105.

Moberg, J. Y., Larsen, D., & Brødsgaard, A. (2017). Striving for balance between caring and restraint: Young adults' experiences with parental multiple sclerosis. *Journal of Clinical Nursing*, *26*, 1363–1374.

Nilsagård, Y., & Boström, K. (2015). Informing the children when a parent is diagnosed as having multiple sclerosis. *International Journal of Multiple Sclerosis Care*, *17*, 42–48.

Özkan, İ, & Polat Dünya, C. (2023). Motherhood experiences of women with multiple sclerosis: A thematic meta-synthesis. *Clinical Nursing Research*, *32*(6), 954–970.

Pakenham, K. I., & Cox, S. (2012). The nature of caregiving in children of a parent with multiple sclerosis from multiple sources and the associations between caregiving activities and youth adjustment overtime. *Psychology and Health*, *7*, 324–346.

Pakenham, K. I., Tilling, J., & Cretchley, J. (2012). Parenting difficulties and resources: The perspectives of parents with multiple sclerosis and their partners. *Rehabilitation Psychology*, *57*, 52–60.

Paliokosta, E., Diareme, S., Kolaitis, G., Ferentinos, S., Lympinaki, E., Tsiantis, J., Romer, G., Karageorgiou, C., Tsiantis, A., Anasontzi, S., & Tsalamanios, E. (2009). Breaking bad news: Communication around parental multiple sclerosis with children. *Families, Systems and Health*, *27*, 64–76.

Payne, D., & McPherson, K. (2010). Becoming mothers. Multiple sclerosis and motherhood: A qualitative study. *Disability and Rehabilitation*, *32*, 629–638.

Prunty, M., Sharpe, L., Butow, P., & Fulcher, G. (2008). The motherhood choice: Themes arising in the decision-making process for women with multiple sclerosis. *Multiple Sclerosis*, *14*, 701–704.

Razaz, N., Nourian, R., Marrie, R. A., Boyce, W. T., & Tremlett, H. (2014). Children and adolescents adjustment to parental multiple sclerosis: A systematic review. *BMC Neurology*, *14*, Article 107.

Rintell, D., & Melito, R. (2013). "Her Illness Is a Project We Can Work on Together". *International Journal of Multiple Sclerosis Care*, *15*, 130–136.

Scabini, E., Lanz, M., & Marta, E. (2006). *Transition to adulthood and family relations: An intergenerational perspective*. Routledge.

Schubert, C., Steinberg, L., Peper, J., Ramien, C., Hellwig, K., Köpke, S., & Rahn, A. C. (2023). Postpartum relapse risk in multiple sclerosis: A systematic review and meta-analysis. *Journal of Neurology, Neurosurgery & Psychiatry*, *94*(9), 718–725.

Starks, H., Morris, M. A., Yorkston, K. M., Johnson, K. L., & Gray, R. F. (2010). Being in- or out-of-sync: Couples' adaptation to change in multiple sclerosis. *Disability and Rehabilitation*, *32*, 196–206.

Strickland, K., Worth, A., & Kennedy, C. (2015). The experiences of support persons of people newly diagnosed with multiple sclerosis: An interpretative phenomenological study. *Journal of Advanced Nursing*, *71*, 2811–2821.

Walsh, F. (1998). *Strenghtening family resilience*. Guilford Press.

Walsh, F. (2016). Family resilience: A developmental systems framework. *European Journal of Developmental Psychology*, *13*, 313–324.

Willson, C. L., Tetley, J., Lloyd, C., Messmer Uccelli, M., & MacKian, S. (2018). The impact of multiple sclerosis on the identity of mothers in Italy. *Disability and Rehabilitation*, *40*, 1456–1467.

Materials and "homework"

Introduction

This appendix contains the handout distributed to the participants in each group containing the materials for each meeting and indications of some activities to be continued individually at home between meetings. This handout constitutes a working tool not only during the meetings, but also afterward: each participant can re-read and re-use it whenever they wish.

This handout can be enriched with suggestive images or graphic photos that refer to the contents gradually addressed in the meetings. Whatever graphic form each person will choose in proposing this type of intervention, we emphasize the need to compose a beautiful, accurate, and attractive handout that enhances the intervention and consequently also the people taking part in it. The inclusion of naturalistic and symbolic photos is particularly recommended.

First meeting

How to do relaxation exercises at home

We can all learn to relax through deep breathing.

A shallow and rapid breathing has negative effects on the functioning of the body, because a lot of stagnant air remains in the lungs. In particular, a rapid and shallow breathing promotes disturbing emotions, such as anxiety, and increases tension and fatigue.

Nature teaches us: we all sigh to de-escalate the tension. To manage emotions such as anxiety, fear, sadness, anger, guilt, shame, and to foster enriching emotions, such as tenderness, affection, joy, gratitude, confidence, serenity, tranquility and calmness, you have to learn to breath and relax.

We can all do this with simple exercises: just repeat the exercises regularly, every day at home.

It is important to make them once a day every day, choosing a quiet moment of the day to your liking and a corner of the house where it's easier not to be disturbed.

When you will have learned to do exercises well and you will be sufficiently trained, you will be able to use this breathing in times of difficulty, when you are angry, anxious, sad, or even during a diagnostic examination or before a visit. You will notice that your body will relax and that your mind will also react in a positive way.

How to learn to relax

Sit comfortably (abandoned arms in your lap, sagging jaw, shoulders released, eyes closed) or lying on the bed (pillow under the head, legs apart, arms stretched and spaced apart from the body, spine stretched out, sagging jaw, shoulders released, eyes closed). Focus on your breathing.

Take fractional breathing: inhale slowly with your nose and count mentally: 1, 2, 3, 4, without throwing the air out every time (for this reason, it is called "fractional breathing"); you'll feel your abdomen rising.

Then exhale slowly by throwing air out of your mouth as if you were blowing into a bottle: you must hear the noise; completely and as much as possible empty your lungs, always counting mentally: 1, 2, 3, 4.

Take 4 fractional breathing: you will notice that each time the breaths will be deeper and that each time the lungs will fill and empty more. As you breathe, imagine your lungs expanding and contracting, like two large sponges.

Continue to breathe deeply and slowly, focusing on your breathing body.

Just listen to your breath.

Then, imagine something that is very pleasant and relaxing for you; images of a meadow, a tree, a flower are useful. Contemplate this image as long as you like to do so. To end, take two deep fractional breathing.

Then, with your eyes closed, move your fingers slowly, then your hands, then stronger: open and close your hands first and then fold your arms; then move your feet and then your legs, first slowly and then strongly, as if to stretch out. Finally, open your eyes again.

Homework

For next time, read the book by Silvia Bonino *Coping with chronic illness. Theories, issues and lived experiences* (London: Routledge, 2021), up to page 23, plus pages 143–145. In this part, the topics we have talked about today are discussed in detail.

Try to describe yourself: who am I?
Three positives of you on a physical level:

① _____

② _____

③ _____

Three positives of you on a psychological level:

① _____

② _____

③ _____

Don't give up the task with the excuse you can't find: there are certainly!

Remember to do relaxation exercises every day, at a suitable time of your choice.

Second meeting

Homework

Remember to do relaxation exercises every day.

Continue reading the book by Silvia Bonino *Coping with chronic illness. Theories, issues and lived experiences* (London: Routledge, 2021), up to page 31, where the topics we have talked about today are discussed in detail.

Write on the paper (only for yourself, you won't be asked to read it during the group session): three things *I would like to change in my life*, to live better:

① _____

② _____

③ _____

Below are the aspects that we discussed in today's meeting, so that you can think back at home, if you wish. What made sense to my life (i.e., it was important, it made me feel fulfilled, I engaged in it, I struggled to get it) before the diagnosis and what changes the diagnosis has introduced. Therefore, *what now gives meaning to my life*.

_____

_____

What could *now give even more meaning to my life*:

1 in affective relationships and family:

_____

_____

2 in friendships:

_____

_____

3 at work:

_____

_____

4 in the community where I live, in my free time:

_____

_____

In concrete terms, **what could I change** to feel that my life is worth living, and therefore to live better?

1 in affective relationships and family:

_____

_____

2 in friendships:

_____

_____

3 at work:

_____

_____

4 in the community where I live, in my free time:

_____

_____

Third meeting

Symptom management

General rules of life

Whatever the symptoms are, some general rules of life must be followed that allow you to feel better.

1 Do not smoke: Smoking is proven to worsen the progression of the disease.

2 Make a healthy diet, that is, rich in vegetables, legumes, cereals, fruits, fish, and low in fat (especially animals), sugar, red meat, sausages and dairy products.

3 Sleep a sufficient number of hours: not too few but not too many. With self-observation, everyone can understand what is the number of hours of sleep that are good for themselves.

4 Do regular exercise, every day, without excess, choosing the activity that you like the most. Avoid both physical scrambles and prolonged inactivity.

5 Avoid alcohol.

How to better manage symptoms

Getting angry or depressed about symptoms of multiple sclerosis doesn't help and just serves to get worse. It is much better to learn how to manage symptoms in the best possible way:

1 Ask health professionals if there are any proven ways that can help you better manage the symptoms you have (e.g., fatigue).

2 Ask your doctor if there are drug therapies that can help you.

3 Try to understand with self-observation what conditions improve or worsen your symptoms.

4 Always with self-observation, try to understand which management strategies are useful to you and which are useless or harmful. Don't forget that each person is different from the other.

5 Don't give up everything that can allow you to do what you want despite the symptoms: various material aids, help from other people, scheduling time and mode of tasks. Try and evaluate what is useful to you or not.

6 Do not be afraid to ask others for help: there is nothing to be ashamed of.

The general principles of energy saving strategies

1 **Balancing activity and rest**: It is important to learn to plan in advance frequent rest times. This allows you to preserve some energy to finish your task and to improve recovery by increasing overall resistance.

2 **Planning your activities**: If you learn to plan in advance your activities, you can distribute workloads to avoid high concentrations. You can alternate between heavy and less demanding activities to avoid excessive fatigue. This planning must be applied to both daily and weekly activities.

3 **Knowing your tolerance and regulating activities**: You must learn, during the execution of the activities, to respect the threshold of fatigue. You must know how to recognize the signs of fatigue early, and to stop before being completely exhausted. This way you will be able to recover more adequately. To this end, it will be important to be able to delegate, to request external support, and to learn to break down the activity at different times.

4 **Establishing priorities**: It is important to learn to reorganize your daily activities based on criteria of importance and satisfaction. Since your energy is easily exhausted, it will be essential to optimize the use of resources by avoiding wasting them on less relevant activities and concentrating instead on the most significant tasks.

5 **Improving the environment**: Making the work environment comfortable reduces energy consumption (e.g., an adequate light fatigues the sight less; air conditioning and ventilated environment improve tolerance; suitable music can help you relax). It is also important to organize the work area by preparing all the tools and materials needed in accessible positions before starting, to facilitate the execution of the activity.

6 **Postural precautions**: It is always necessary to work in favorable positions, in order to avoid energy waste (when possible carry out sitting activities) and overloads (incorrect postures). In this sense, it is appropriate to study the ergonomics of the movements and follow the indications of postural hygiene.

7 **Use of aids**: They reduce energy consumption and simplify the task by increasing the autonomy (example: crutch to improve balance and walking, household appliances and home shopping service to reduce fatigue and time devoted to houseworks, portable diaries to facilitate attention and memory, and alarms on the phone to remember appointments, taking medicines, etc.).

8 **Learning to relax**: With relaxation techniques, management of rest times, deep, and fractionated breathing.

9 **Curing sleep**: Sleeping a subjectively optimal number of hours, eliminating as much as possible the disturbing factors (noise, heat, poor digestion, physical discomfort, etc.).

Homework

Remember to do relaxation exercises every day.

For next time, continue reading the book by Silvia Bonino *Coping with chronic illness. Theories, issues and lived experiences* (London: Routledge, 2021), up to page 83, where the topics we have talked about today are discussed in detail.

What **goals** are or could be **important and meaningful to me but at the same time achievable** (possibly changing the ones I had)? Here are the steps and questions you need to ask yourself to achieve your goals in the following areas:

1 in affective relationships and family:

_____

_____

2 in friendships:

_____

_____

3 at work:

_____

_____

4 in the community where I live, in my free time:

_____

_____

What *precise strategies* can allow me to achieve my goal?

_____

_____

How can I *evaluate my behavior and make the necessary adjustments*?

_____

_____

Fourth meeting

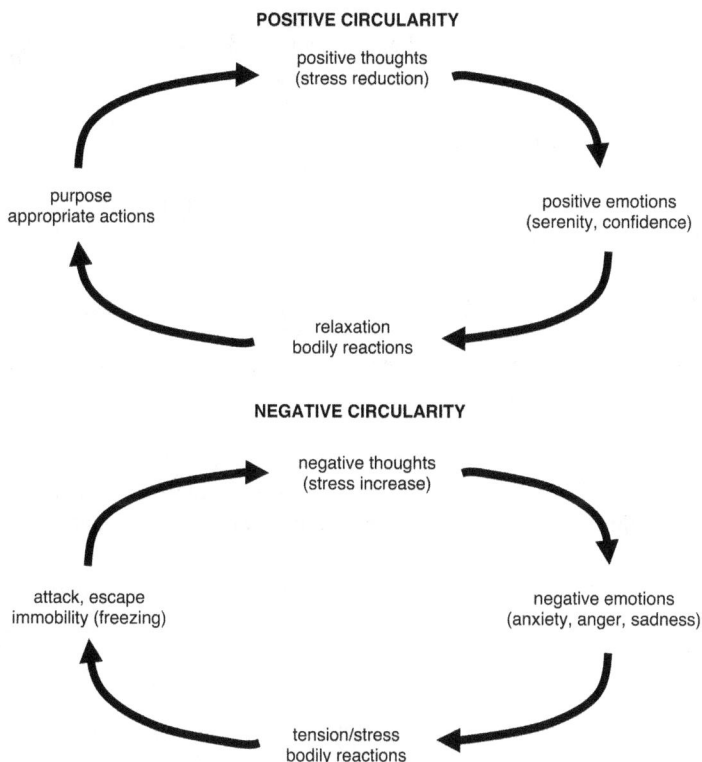

POSITIVE CIRCULARITY

positive thoughts
(stress reduction)

positive emotions
(serenity, confidence)

relaxation
bodily reactions

purpose
appropriate actions

NEGATIVE CIRCULARITY

negative thoughts
(stress increase)

negative emotions
(anxiety, anger, sadness)

tension/stress
bodily reactions

attack, escape
immobility (freezing)

From thoughts to emotions: Thoughts can increase or reduce stress

The following examples help you understand how thoughts can promote discomfort or well-being:

Negative thought: I've been diagnosed with MS: my life is over
Illusory thought: I am invincible: MS can't do anything against me.
Positive thought: I have MS, but I'm still able to do many things, like for example…

Negative thought: With MS there is no future
Illusory thought: Just don't think about anything
Positive thought: I can find the way to do what is important for me, for example I can…

Negative thought: I broke dishes again: I'm no longer able to do anything
Illusory thought: It is important that no one knows!
Positive thought: Patience! Breaking dishes is not so bad: it can happen to everyone, even those who do not have MS.

Negative thought: I fell again: I am now an incapable
Illusory thought: Who cares!
Positive thought: Luckily this time I didn't get hurt. But I have to find a way to stop falling: changing course, changing shoes, leaning on someone…

Negative thought: I can't do this things as well as I used to
Illusory thought: Nothing has changed and I can do everything as before
Positive thought: I do this activity as best I can. If it has any flaws, patience. The important thing is that I did it!

Negative thought: I'm not able to do this activity
Illusory thought: I can do everything!
Positive thought: If I organize in the right way, I can do it. I have confidence in my chances

Negative thought: It bothers me when people look at me
Illusory thought: That people look at me is completely indifferent to me
Positive thought: I don't have to think bad. I also happen to look at others

Do this exercise: compare your thoughts with the examples and decide if they are negative, illusory or positive thoughts. If they are negative or illusory, try to change them in positive thoughts.

Small rules to manage emotions that are a source of suffering and encourage positive ones

1   Learn to relax through breathing exercises, in calm moments, daily and regularly; you can imagine calm, pleasant and relaxing situations. Everybody can learn to relax: you have to regularly repeat these exercises. After you've trained well, use these exercises to reduce tension at critical moments.

2   Pay attention to your body to understand what emotion you are experiencing: fear, anxiety, anger, sadness, joy, excitement, …

3   Try to write down the physical sensations (compulsion/lightness in the chest, knot/lightness in the throat, tension/softness in the stomach, etc.). Talk to a trusted person, too.

4   When you experience an emotion that creates suffering, ask yourself what caused it. Once you have focused the problem, imagine all possible solutions and eliminate non-viable ones. Finally, choose the solution that feels best for you. Evaluate it after a certain time, to change or confirm it.

5 Don't brood over what's missing in your life if it's not in your power to procure: it only serves to get depressed and feel bad. Focus your attention on what you have of positive and value it: thoughts can change emotions.

6 Do not mull over the past, about how you acted, about events that happened, about the wrongs suffered... the past cannot be changed and this rumination has the sole effect of feeling bad and increasing anger and depression. Blocking negative thoughts is possible.

7 Ask yourself if what you are worried about is under your control or not. Don't worry about things that are not under your control; instead invest energy on the things that are. Most of the concerns for the future will thus come to fall, because it concerns aspects that cannot be controlled by us.

8 Identify situations that are positive, relaxing, fun, enjoyable and achievable for you. Everyone has their own: think about it and you will find them. Find moments during the day and the week to make room for these pleasant moments: nothing and no one can stop you.

9 Listen to music that is suitable for relaxing, not syncopated or percussive. For example, classical music is very useful in this regard and in particular that of Mozart has shown that it is able to provide well-being. In any case, choose melodies that have a relaxing effect on you.

10 Try to look at reality with an ironic eye. Learn to laugh at yourself too, without taking yourself too seriously.

Homework

Remember to do relaxation exercises every day.

For next time, continue reading the book by Silvia Bonino *Coping with chronic illness. Theories, issues and lived experiences* (London: Routledge, 2021) until the end.

Do the exercise "From thoughts to emotions: thoughts can increase or reduce stress".

Fifth meeting

Learning to ask others for help (family, friends, colleagues)

1 Tell others clearly if and when you want their help (for example, to give you the arm, to accompany you, etc.). Others cannot know our desires unless we tell them clearly. They also often fear being intrusive and inappropriate: this is why they do not come forward and do not offer to help us.

2 Do not consider a decrease in your value asking for help from others to perform certain tasks. Giving up a goal so as not to ask anyone for help is an excess of pride, wrong and counterproductive. In fact, it turns against us, so that we cannot do what we would like. It is not a question of "lowering" oneself to ask, but of evaluating who, how, when and under what conditions can help us. What matters is to reach the goal that interests us.

3 Consider how to reciprocate others for their help, if this is important to you; remember that there are not only economic and material rewards. However, with gratitude you also accept free help and do not feel diminished by it: on the contrary, the attention of others is a sign of your value.

Rules of good communication with others (family, friends, colleagues)

1 Clearly say what you want or do not want: others cannot know if we do not tell them. It is too demanding to ask them to guess our desires from our expression, our behavior or our silences.

2 Do not hide your thoughts, opinions, desires, hoping that others will ask you for them. It only serves to feel bad, to feel misunderstood and sad. Others may have many reasons for not asking: shyness, modesty, fear of hurting, anxiety. Their silence does not in itself mean superficiality, disinterest or refusal.

3 Do not use ambiguous formulations (example: "Monday I need the car to go to the hospital because I have no one accompanying me", instead of "Monday I go to the hospital and I'd like you to accompany me") which can be interpreted in different ways. They put others in difficulty, because they don't know how to do it, and they turn against us, because they are the cause of misunderstanding.

4 Above all, take advantage of moments of calm to talk about yourself and your needs: at times when you are angry you risk saying things badly. In any case, it is better to say even sharply what is important for us rather than not talking about it at all

Rules of self-observation

1 Carefully observe what happens in your body and put it in writing; just a simple agenda on which you write your observations, every week or even every day, if you consider it necessary.

2 Keep a diary for new, more disturbing or uncontrollable symptoms. The diary is essential to understand if there are regularities, antecedent situations to be avoided as harmful or to be favored because they are useful. This will make it easier for you to discuss it with the healthcare staff. It is not enough to trust the memory: you can be wrong.

Rules of communication with healthcare professionals

1 Always ask when you have questions or concerns, and if it is not clear, ask again. Don't say "yes" if you don't understand, not to disturb or for fear of looking "stupid". The patient has the right to ask and the doctor and nurse have the duty to always reply.

2 Ask to write down the prescriptions (how to do a therapy, how many times, how, etc.). Everyone can forget and mistakes can have very serious consequences. In self-administered therapies, keep a diary where you can record your reactions, so that you can communicate them to your health care professional. Even in this case, a simple agenda is enough to write down one's observations.

Homework

Remember to do relaxation exercises every day.

Continue to refer to the book by Silvia Bonino *Coping with chronic illness. Theories, issues and lived experiences* (London: Routledge, 2021) by rereading the parts that interest you.

Keep the following steps in mind when planning something:

i ask yourself which goals are important and meaningful, but at the same time reachable;

ii ask yourself what strategies, tools or aids can be useful to achieve these goals and

iii evaluate the result and make the necessary adjustments.

Do every week the exercise "From thoughts to emotions: thoughts can increase or reduce stress".

Reread every week all the material you have been given on the management of physical symptoms, emotions and communication.

Sixth meeting - Follow-up

Here are some suggestions for the coming months.

Remember to do relaxation exercises every day.

When planning something, keep the following steps in mind:

- ask yourself which goals are important and meaningful but at the same time achievable;
- ask yourself which strategies, tools or aids can enable you to achieve these goals and
- then evaluate the result and make the necessary adjustments.

Reread all the material you have been given on the management of physical symptoms, emotions and communication.

Do each week the exercise "From thought to emotions: thoughts can increase or reduce stress" (fourth meeting).

Continue to refer to the book by Silvia Bonino *Coping with chronic illness. Theories, issues and lived experiences* (London: Routledge, 2021), rereading the parts that most interest you.

The words of the participants

First meeting: The group and identity

Examples of feelings experienced at diagnosis and expressed through images

- I chose the image of a terrified face wearing a white mask.
- I chose the image of a dandelion. It feels like the pistils of a dandelion.
- "I feel fragile". Just one breath and you feel like you're falling apart.

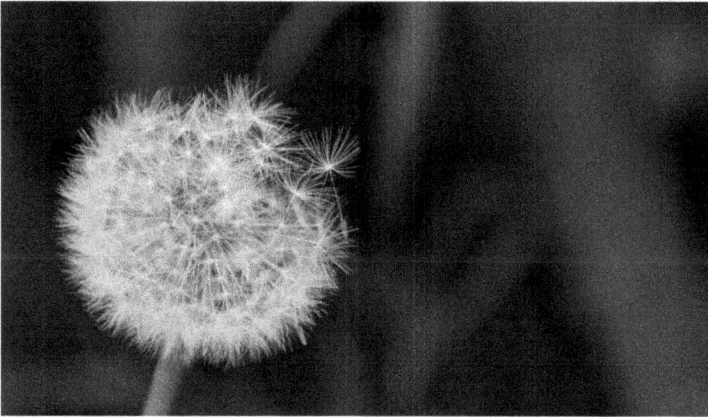

- I also chose a snowy landscape with fog to symbolize a future that I perceive as unclear, unstable and changing.
- I chose the image of a swimmer. At first, I felt a strong sense of disbelief. At first, I felt crushed, as if I lived under the bed all day. But just like a swimmer who keeps her head under water for a short time and then re-emerges into the light, now I am facing the disease with positivity.
- I chose the image of a landscape with fog because I have the feeling of walking in the fog and because you can see in this image a man with his shoulders hunched, helpless, whose only possibility is to accept his condition. I felt helpless, sad and with little hope for the future.

- I chose the image of a freediver. During the interview with the neurologist I felt like I was freediving, I didn't expect it. The second image is a landscape covered in fog that symbolizes confusion ("Oh my God, how do I organize myself? What do I do with my son?").
- The image that represents the disease is that of a boxer, the diagnosis came like a blow, a punch in the face. The other image is that of a landscape covered in fog that represents my lack of understanding of the disease (I don't know what it is, nor what's behind it).

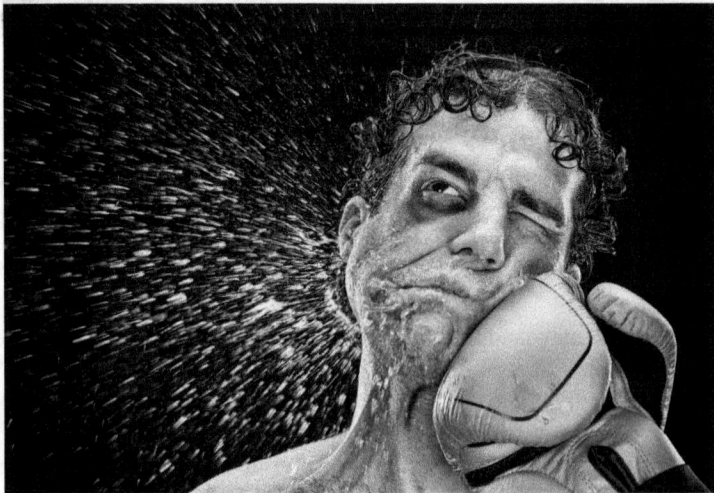

- I chose the image of a mountain. This place is inhospitable and represents illness, but there are other people in the distance who are in the same condition. I don't think this place is so bad because it has to be looked at from the right point of view. In fact, there is snow and you can therefore ski even if it is cold.

- The diagnosis was like a bolt from the blue, a shoe that crushed me to the ground. I felt crushed when I was diagnosed with multiple sclerosis following paresthesia and mobility problems. The hospitalization was made easier by my being a nurse, but on the other hand knowing what was happening to me led me to great fear because I feared I had ALS. Fear was the predominant emotion until the moment of the diagnosis, then confusion set in as I do not have much neurological knowledge. By switching to the patient's side, I was able to experience the feeling of cortisone withdrawal and understand what it means to be on the other side. In the end, this diagnosis is an opportunity for change for me.

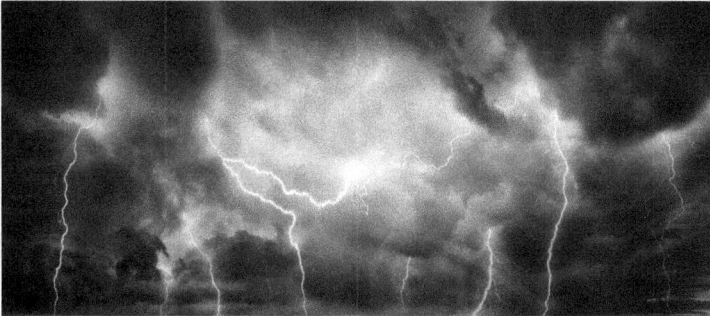

- I feel a strong sense of clarity. I chose the image of a white ball breaking a triangle of billiard balls. From May to December of last year, I had no certainty and I found the wait very difficult. The confirmation of the diagnosis thanks to the tests was a liberation because it defined what the problem was. I felt a sense of pleasantness and clarity, which for me is a starting point.
- For me, the image of a person alone in the middle of the sea represents the sensations of loneliness and confusion.
- The image of a cliff expresses how, emotionally, I felt everything falling apart.
- I chose the image of a frightened little animal and an amphora in the middle of the sea. I immediately felt a sense of apnea and heaviness, isolation (amphora). Although I am still going through the phase of disbelief, I think it is better to accept this condition, but I still feel a strong inner isolation, I feel an isolated landscape inside me, and I still struggle to accept reality.

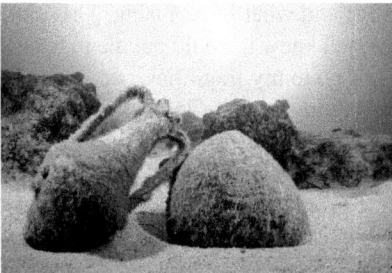
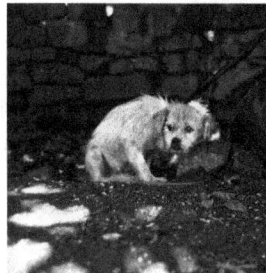

- I choose the image of the desert because at the time of diagnosis I felt alone and doomed, "like having a tumor in the final stage". The hastiness and lack of sensitivity on the part of the medical team contributed in part to the feeling of bewilderment.

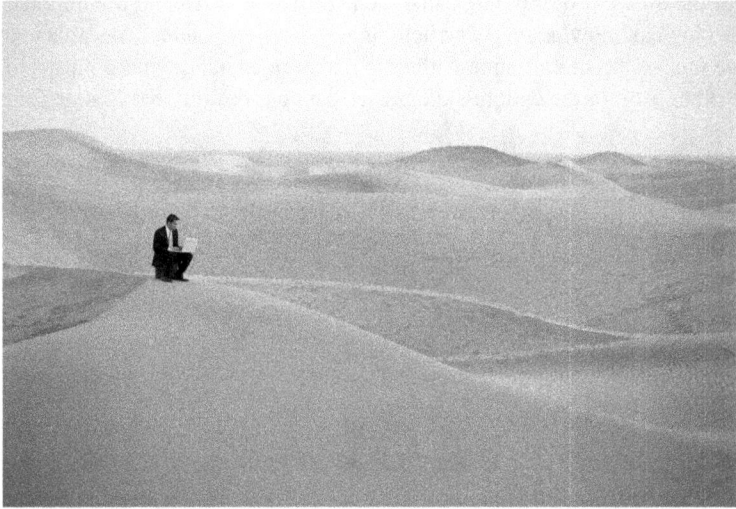

- The first image chosen is a field of tulips for two reasons: on the one hand, I feel lucky because while I was hospitalized I had around me people who were much younger, but at the same time on the horizon, there is a cycling path that I see as the path I have to face with the disease. The second image is a mountain that I feel I have to climb to the top. I want to fight for my future.
- I felt that I was helpless because I couldn't even blame myself. I felt like I was in the open sea, far out, without even a life jacket.
- For me, the image is this dangerous road sign with a car skidding because for me it was the end of the world, I would never have expected it. "Why me?" I trace the image back to an episode in which the car blocked an intersection, and my legs were blocked too.
- For me, the night image of a mountain with a full moon. The mountain, which in this moment symbolizes the cycle of encounters, has a positive function because it can put me in touch with what I love and what I fear losing. This path scared me and I was reluctant to take it because I knew it would put me in front of emotions, fueling the fear of letting myself go to my fragilities.
- The image of the sea, with some birds flying together in the sky, symbolizes the feeling I felt when I was diagnosed. I felt like the ground was disappearing from under my feet, but I thought I could do it alone and that I didn't need help, so much so that I refused the invitation to group meetings. Now, after a year, I have realized that I have to start "flying low" and I am happy that I am not alone in facing the disease.

- I chose the image of a shoe because I am afraid that the disease could take away my ability to walk, run, and be independent.
- I chose the image of a smile because at the moment of the diagnosis I had a moment of relief, I thought it was something more serious. In fact, in my family everyone predicted terrible things for me.
- I felt as alone as the image of this mountain, also because it is alone that one faces the disease. I chose it both because it is what I saw in front of me at the moment of diagnosis, and because I immediately stopped mountaineering, no longer trusting my body.

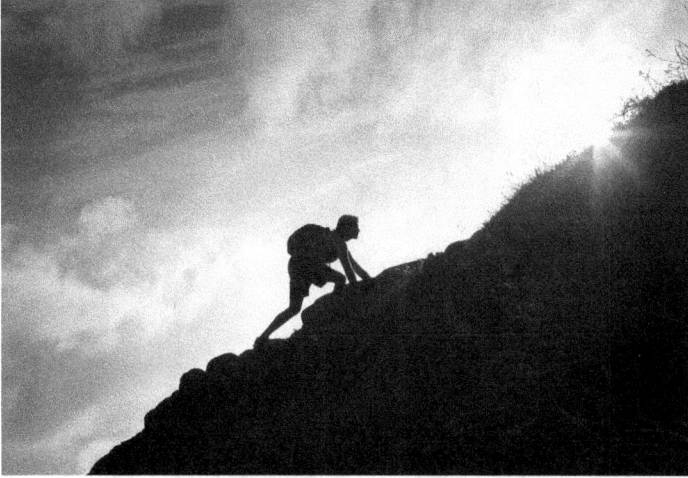

- I chose the car that skids. I have always tried to define a precise line of professional and family goals that I should pursue to achieve my personal happiness, but at the time of the diagnosis everything I was trying to build faltered.

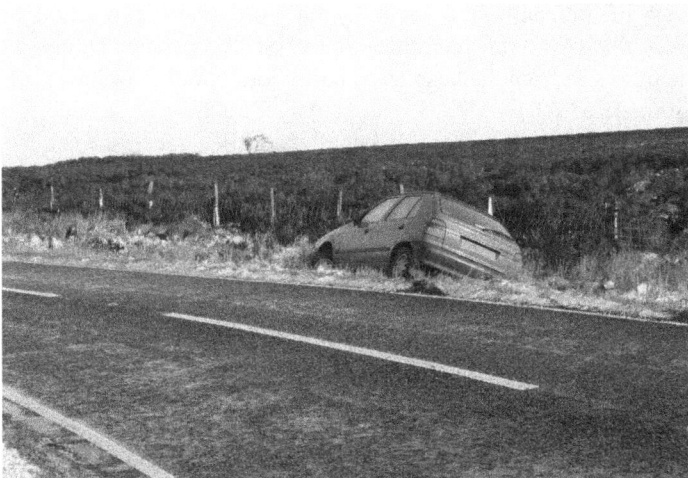

Freezing examples

- It's like a fog has descended, I can't see anything anymore. My brother had multiple sclerosis and passed away some time ago, so I knew what it was, so I had this reaction.
- I'm like dead; after the diagnosis I just wanted to be alone, I closed myself off.
- I feel the cold. Since I received the diagnosis, it is as if everything was stopped, blocked and frozen.

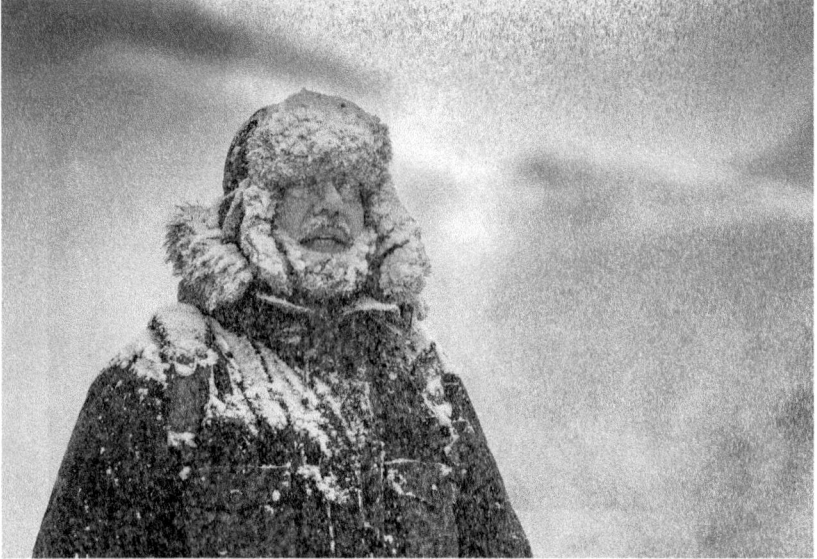

Examples of struggle

- I face my life rationally so I would say that I had a rational reaction, I rationalized everything by putting emotions aside a bit. The constant thought I had during the tram ride from the hospital to home was: "Well, now how do I face the trip to America?".
- The world immediately fell on me, but after a while I got up and understood that I have to face it.
- I didn't take the news of the diagnosis too badly because I had known for years that something was wrong and I had been undergoing continuous tests; in fact, when I heard the news, I replied: "Well, what do we do now?!". What broke my heart was the fact that multiple sclerosis had effectively blocked my search for a pregnancy: I was living a happy moment, the right one, and for the moment I had to put aside the idea of becoming a mother, which for me represents a strong desire.

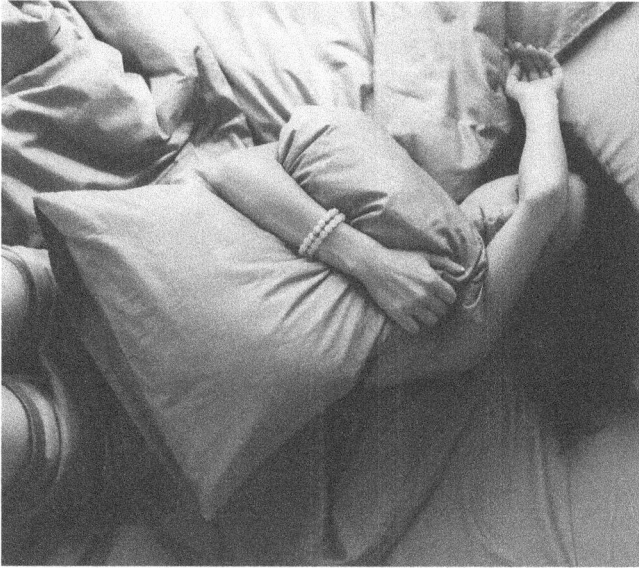

Examples of avoidance

- I have to think about the here and now; I have always been calm, I have to see more in the long term, I got angry at the diagnosis, then I felt indifferent. My mood has ups and downs. I have to help my parents take it as a "game", I made others understand that the disease is not something I have, it is in my body, but it is not mine, I do what I want with myself.
- The image I chose represents a woodpecker that takes refuge in a trunk, and it refers to an ostrich that hides its head in the sand to push away the thought of the disease by pretending it is not there.
- My reaction to the diagnosis was, "Who cares! Let's move on!".

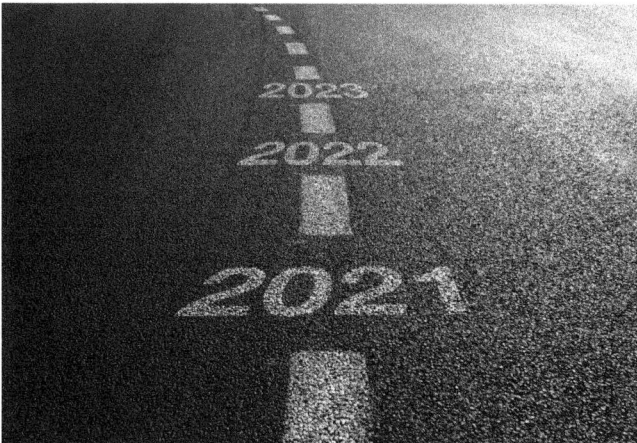

- I chose the spider web, because the first time I was sick I couldn't do anything, while in my head I could do everything, and I felt trapped in my own body. After the diagnosis, I started not caring about anything, even my health. After that, it got better.

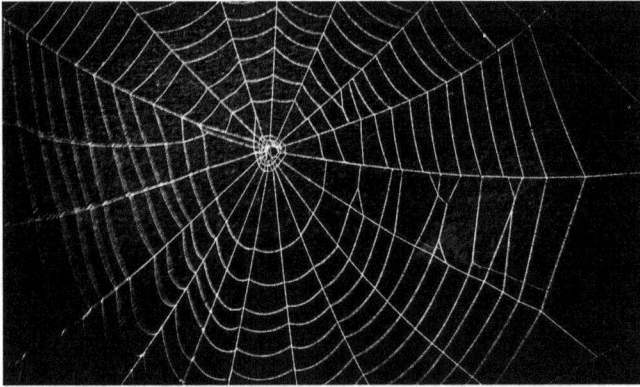

Examples of feelings experienced in the present, in the here, and now

- I chose the image of two eyes that peer, which symbolize my attempt to understand the disease.
- I chose the image of a character in balance, leaning on a fragile structure with all the possible body parts. The situation is still unclear and I don't know where it will take me. Even though I'm 48, it's better that it happened to me rather than to younger people, but I still feel this sensation of being in balance ("But if it hadn't happened to me, even better!"). All in all, however, I can do what I like, so I'm positive.
- I chose the image of a river flowing with reeds carried by the current. I feel dragged by the disease because, being a planner, after the diagnosis I felt like I had to say "Okay, try not to plan everything for yourself and for others, but limit yourself to one little piece at a time".
- I feel like a cheetah waiting but I still don't know if I'm hunter or prey. The prevailing sensation is one of firmness and immobility.

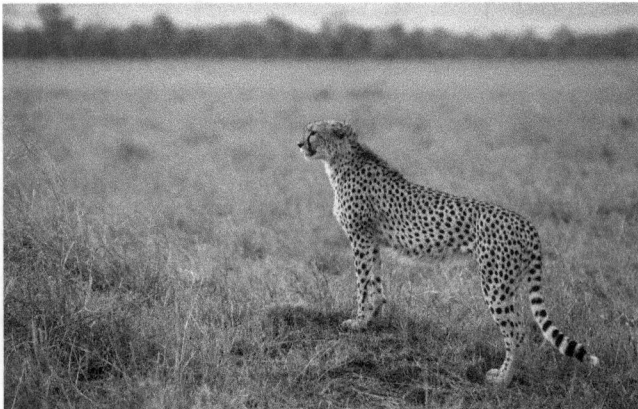

- I chose the image of a motorcyclist slowed down by mud and splashes. I would like to go at full speed, but I feel tired and I get splashed and get stuck with the bike, so I have to slow down. Being a planner, with the diagnosis I was forced to change. At the moment, I feel subjected to a lot of stress because I don't know how to take things as they come.
- I chose the image of a natural landscape seen from the glass of a window. This is representative of my need for calm and tranquility, to be able to carve out time and moments for myself, but on the other hand I don't want to close myself off from the world. The glass is seen as a division from the world external but it can open at any time. At the moment I feel like a passive spectator who watches from inside the room, but my will is to absolutely not lose contact with the world and nature.
- I chose as the first image a landscape with fog in which I feel immersed, wrapped. A second image is of a laboratory, which recalls my work environment. There are some plants in small test tubes that are growing (regrowth) but that need to be looked after (reorganizing one's life). I have to learn to take better care of myself, even those around me. I am looking for a balance and I am still in a state of confusion and fear. I am anxious for fear that the situation of the first hospitalization will repeat itself, breaking my routine.

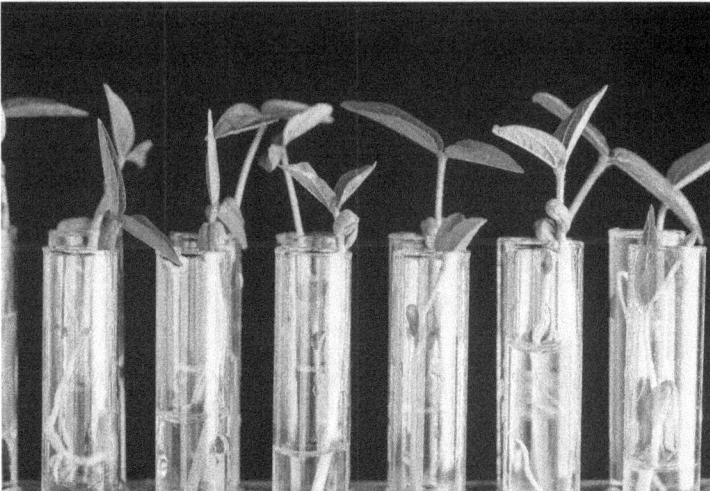

- I feel like this flower among many dandelions in a field. After the diagnosis, not having much information about the disease, I felt without any reference points. On the other hand, thanks to multiple sclerosis, I have tripled my circle of friends, now I feel part of a group where everyone is doing something with me.
- I chose the image of lightning, they represent the attacks of the disease. I have many desires, including that of opening my own company, but there are many difficulties that prevent me, both financial and health-related. This makes me

feel like a little girl watching the storm. I cannot choose not to face this situation, I am worried about my future for the people around me and as I said before also for my boyfriend.

- I chose the image of a cheetah on a tree, I feel out of place like this animal in the image, I want to go back to being like before, I want to go back to being who I am, I struggle to explain what I mean, and I have difficulty adapting to new needs.
- I chose the image of buffaloes climbing a mountain; now I feel more combative, despite the difficulties that I will surely encounter during the climb I have no intention of giving up.
- I also chose the image of the "climb", of penguins climbing a glacier, for the exact same reason.
- I chose the image of the woods on the water, because even today I feel tied, dragged by events. I have liver problems, and my biggest worry for now is whether I will have to take the drug for life.
- I chose the image of three climbers roped together representing past, present and future. The moment of administering the drug three times a week represents a break from daily life. Today I am more aware, but not happy knowing that I have to follow the therapy. My goal is to get higher, to the first climber represented in the image. Being a planner by nature, the disease, which is not plannable, is not easily accepted because it is perceived as unknown. In the past I have been mourning the loss of the person I loved. The future is the prospect of being able to tolerate even the unknown, trying to live day by day and being more carefree.

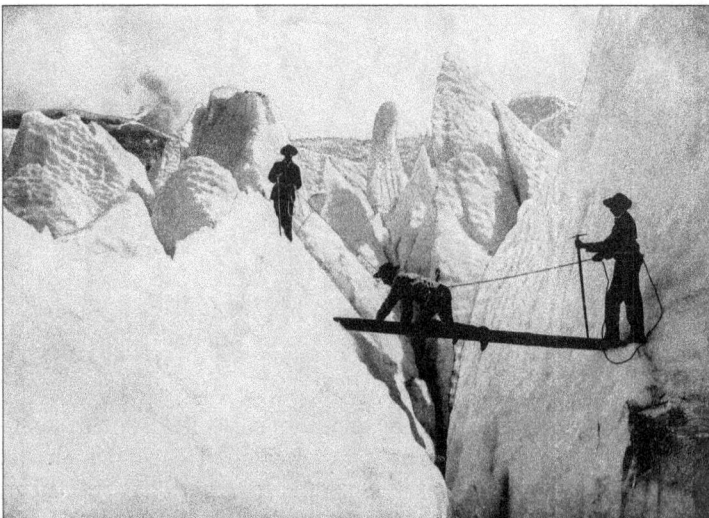

- I chose two images, one represents "turning the page" and the other a winding river. I have to face the disease, and that's also why I'm here today, I want to do something but I feel blocked, now I want to start. The road I have to travel is like this winding river, it's long because it's full of curves, but I have to travel it to get where I want, I have to do something.

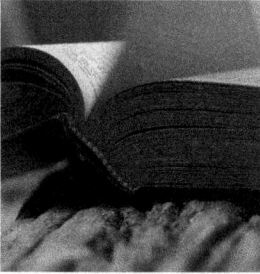

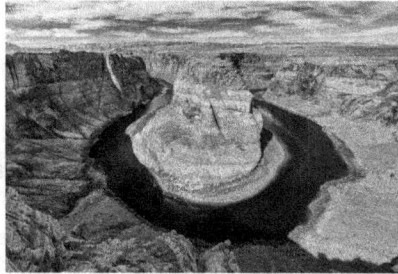

- I chose the image of the sea with clouds, even if I don't feel fully reflected. I am there, the disease too, but I want and I am stronger than those "clouds". My head is very important to me, and right now I don't want to think about "this thing"; I think there are worse things. I have a different situation than others, I'm 60, I'm single, but that doesn't mean I don't have my loved ones. I still want to consider myself lucky.
- I chose the image, a little blurry, of the running lion: for me it represents life that passes quickly. There's no point in stopping to think, there's no point in playing the victim.
- I chose the image of the sunset over the sea, which is not who I am but what I would like to be. I know I'm no longer as sunny as I used to be.
- I chose the image that most resembled "paths". I love to travel, in fact I left three days after starting the drug. I managed to walk despite the pain, perhaps because I have a very high pain threshold.
- I will try to adapt the image I chose to my thoughts. For me, the future is a huge black hole, it has always been even before the illness because of my precarious job. I feel "heavy" as during a climb that I am afraid to start. The illness has "blocked" me even more than I was before.
- I chose the image of a black and white mask that reminds me of myself at the time of the diagnosis. I felt infinite sadness and the thought of death tormented me. The news changed every perspective. It's only been four months since the diagnosis, it's still a hard blow.
- I chose the image that represents the edge of the precipice. That's how I felt. I found out I had multiple sclerosis two years ago, when my baby girl was about to be born. When I received the confirmation, it was a void for me. The first week was hard, I was in a lot of crisis, then I recovered but it's as if I had become emotionally numb. My idea of multiple sclerosis was to end up in a wheelchair.
- I chose the image of a forest where there is only a small "square" in the middle; there I am, alone with my fears. Once upon a time if I got a tingling sensation I didn't worry about it, now I'm terrified of it, perhaps because I feel immersed in this "gigantic forest" that I don't know, there is no path that I know I can take.

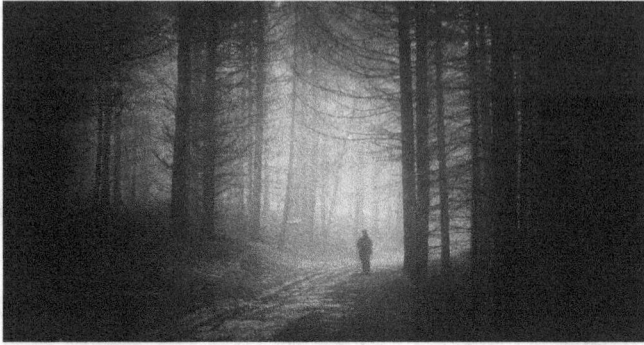

- I chose an image with electrical wires, but I imagine them more tangled than that. The situation is intricate and I have to find a way to untangle that tangle. I had a strong reaction at the beginning, then I tried to take it philosophically and I arrived at CReSM. It was a sudden blow, then there was a settling in with some more ups and downs.
- I chose the image of dandelions because thanks to the meeting I feel like I have blown away the negative part of the disease, perhaps I am a little reassured by the experiences of others.
- I chose a person who enters a fortress because I am ashamed and fear social judgment, so isolation in the "fortress" has a protective function for me.
- I choose the course of this river that flows and is master of its own spaces, eroding the ground or retreating to change course (a bit like the omnipotence of the writer, who decides who to let live and how).
- I chose the image of a ballerina jumping in a meadow. As usual I am different from the others, I chose this image because for me the diagnosis was a sigh of relief, an answer I had been waiting for a long time. Years ago I started suffering from epilepsy, I am drug resistant and I could not find a cure and an explanation for this discomfort. When I was diagnosed with multiple sclerosis everything became clearer. The worst was after. I was not worried about myself but about those who would be close to me. I told my boyfriend that he was not obliged to live with me, that he was free.

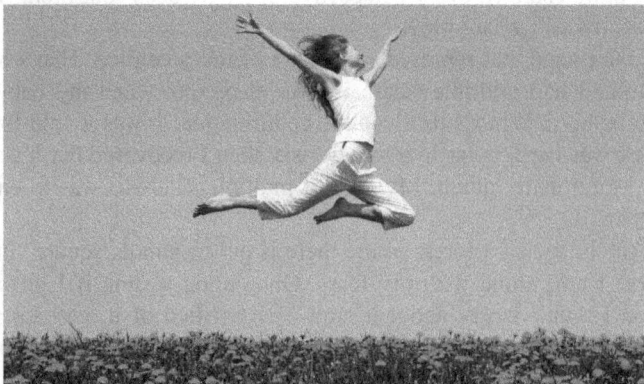

Second meeting – identity and objectives

Examples of responses to the theme of projects and goals that give meaning to life

Who says nothing has changed since the diagnosis

- My "watershed" between a before and after diagnosis coincides with the back problems that began years before the multiple sclerosis. My wife has always been a friend to me and we spend every free moment together walking and going on Sunday trips. As for friends, I sometimes see them for barbecues in the garden or to go out together, but basically nothing has changed. I haven't told anyone that I have multiple sclerosis, not even my daughter, only my wife knows. I would like to be able to tell my daughter that I am ill, but I can't because I feel blocked. I haven't noticed any particular changes coinciding with the diagnosis, as for years in my life back pain has led me to do different activities and limit the ones I used to do.
- I am angry but this is my nature. No one knows about my illness except my husband and my son, I deny it because I don't want to be pitied. I meditate and breathe to get rid of the plaques. There hasn't been a change because I refuse the illness. Who tells me that the symptoms I have aren't brought on by menopause? Maybe the diagnosis is wrong, medicine isn't perfect. I have had conflicting medical opinions and I have accepted the least painful.

Who says that everything has changed and nothing makes sense anymore

- I am a bit resigned, I admit that I am unable to set or see future goals for myself, because just when I made an important change in my life by changing jobs, setting myself new goals and new conquests to achieve, the illness arrived.

Who is aware of their attempts at change

- The meaning for me today is to live fully day by day, to live with love, to love oneself but also others, not giving weight to certain "useless" things. I am constantly changing, I can only make plans from one week to the next, but that doesn't mean I don't dedicate my days to my hobbies: I paint, I walk, I live. It's strange to stay at home so much, but I'm positive, even if I had to say no to soccer games with friends, no to walks in the mountains. I've opened a new expectation on life: I'm looking for more sensitivity, more fullness. There's too much time wasted getting angry, we need to change our attitude, and I'm doing it.
- In my free time, I volunteer with disabled kids. I have managed not to let the disease enter as violently as in other fields, it is the part of my life in which multiple sclerosis has entered less and in which I feel most fulfilled. Compared to university, I have discovered that it will be able to offer me job opportunities here too and not just abroad, so I feel more at peace because I would like to continue to be treated in Italy. The area that has been most affected by the disease is

that of emotional relationships. My goal would be to be able to accept the fact that others will never be able to fully understand me.

- I used to be a beautician, but giving massages became tiring and I had to change jobs. However, I have tried to keep this dimension as an activity to do in my free time, the meaning I have attributed to it has changed. For example, sometimes we meet up with my friends to get my nails done.

- I decided to dedicate myself a little more to myself. I take a closer look at myself, I no longer feel guilty if I give up an outing because I want to stay home. I started to give more importance to what makes me feel good. I pay more attention to selecting friends and understanding what a certain person can give me. In my family, perhaps we love each other more. I no longer complain about stupid things and I often think "What a beautiful family". In general, I try to optimize my resources by using them in what makes me feel good.

- I found this trick: since Interferon doesn't let me sleep, after having the injection I start watching the TV series I like together with my husband. This way I don't make it just Interferon time.

- I have a full life, I always thought that children grow up and that I could have little time for myself. Now the feeling is that having multiple sclerosis could and should be an additional stimulus to demand this space. If before I had a thousand excuses, now is the right time to carve out some space for myself.

- Paradoxically, I feel happier now than before. The carefree attitude is gone forever and I gave him the funeral, but multiple sclerosis is a bomb that has swept away what was not solid. Now I have the stubbornness to say that as long as I'm well I have many things to do and I want to do other things. I am very energetic mentally and I have to accept that the pace slows down. Before I was a crazy pinball that ran. Now, even though I know there is a dark cloud, I know the cloud is there but it is not me.

- Graduating, starting a family, having a baby, are the same things I wanted before, only now I want to do them faster.

- I'm making my pregnancy happen; the diagnosis gave me certainty, in a certain sense I was already prepared, the period before was worse, the one waiting for the diagnosis, when no one knew what I had.

- My baby was born right before the diagnosis, and I have to do everything I can to be well, for him.

- I need to plan, now I'm thinking about a pregnancy; I want to keep my planning in the various areas with the disease as a "new friend".

- I've taken up botany, gardening.

- I go to flea markets with my sister.

- I go to the gym and dance, they are activities that bring me into contact with the body; I also started making bread, I like the idea of eating something made by me, I organize my day based on the times it takes to prepare the bread. One aspect that perhaps is transversal to all areas is that I seek contact with nature, I need to be outdoors, sometimes I want to change my life, go and live in a cabin in the mountains.

- I travel.

- I dedicate myself to my "creations", I make candles, it gives me satisfaction to make them and give them as gifts.
- I feel the need to focus more on myself, also seeking the help of my family, in the division of activities, if necessary. I considered buying a ground floor house considering it a good investment.
- I face what will come tomorrow with a different spirit. I can no longer have the hyperactivity of before, so everything has changed. However, this made me discover how I had underestimated certain feelings (love and friendship) that now I see in the right proportion. I appreciate the real things in life, when you are strong and everything is going well you don't give it weight. I enjoy the little things to the fullest.
- I haven't noticed any major changes compared to before. Now I'm realizing myself in my children, one will soon have to enter the world of work, the other will choose high school, so I like to help them in their choices. I also want to invest in everyday life, do everything I have to, from work to housework. When I was given cortisone I couldn't do anything anymore, now I appreciate the strength I have to do things. I also had a psychological breakdown, in fact I'm taking an antidepressant. My family has given me a lot of support, especially my husband and my sister. My husband replaced me in managing the family when I was sick, he was close to me physically and psychologically and is very involved.
- In my free time I really like to dedicate myself to the house, I live and take care of it more also with the prospect of sharing it with my boyfriend in the future. The goal I have set myself is to dedicate myself more to the house with a view to living it better. Compared to work, I experienced the return a little badly because I didn't know how to handle any questions about my condition. Now I am a little more prepared to answer you in kind, I have learned to defend myself in a good way. I have realized that at work when I am not there, my absence is felt: I feel I am worthy and I am very pleased. Before I thought I was replaceable. This helps me to worry less about a future absence for maternity leave, I feel that I deserve it and that I should not condition my private life based on work.
- Since the diagnosis I have allowed myself to work a little less. I am trying to focus my energies on trying to understand what I want from a work point of view. I am trying to optimize the time I work in order to then be able to give myself breaks. On Saturdays I take care of the house and the shopping, on Sundays I get the shot, so I cut myself off from activities that I used to do. Until recently, Sundays were dedicated to self-injection, but now I'm starting to understand that I can carve out short moments to do something I like.

Examples of dysfunctional attitudes related to illness

- I try not to find out, I don't want to know anything, I try to deny the disease. The therapy upsets me a lot, it disturbs me. For me, the fact of being here is a big step. I decided that I had to do something for myself, because undergoing therapy every day sent me into a crisis.

- The disease is not my thing, it's in my body, but it's not mine, I do what I want with myself. I find another way to do what I like. It's not my thing, let's not talk about something I have. If I think like that, about how I'll be tomorrow, I feel bad. When I go for therapy, I don't think about going to the hospital, I think about going to see other people, and so every relapse is experienced in a less serious way. This thing, as it came, must go away. I don't want there to be a meaning to the disease.
- I changed its name, because "words do things": I call it "my characteristic", not the disease or multiple sclerosis.
- After the diagnosis I feel like I'm in a tunnel that I associate with a sense of injustice, sadness and discouragement linked to thinking "It's not my life, it's not happening to me".

Examples of functional attitudes related to illness

- The disease has also helped me to focus on myself, I ended a relationship that devastated me. I learned to ski, something I always wanted to do.
- I have to thank this disease in part, because it has allowed me to dedicate more time to myself. Representing a bigger problem than a devastating romantic relationship, it gave me the strength to leave it. I still feel very lonely, because I live alone. I didn't want to involve my parents in the visits.
- Compared to before, I need to do relaxing activities. I learned to knit, it relaxes me a lot and helps me to clear my mind, I only focus on that. Before, however, I aimed for much more lively activities.
- Compatible with everyone's schedules, I try to make time to go to the pool or the gym. However, I allow myself to be a little lazier, if I don't feel like going once I don't do it. Before, on the other hand, I didn't. On the weekend, my free time is based on my children, but it's still pleasant.
- I would like to recover my relationship and move in with my partner. I had put this desire aside following the diagnosis because I was afraid of not being able to do it, of always needing my mother's care. Now, however, I am putting this thought to the side and am determined to reach my goal.

Third meeting – symptom management

Energy saving strategies

- It helps me to try to feel my breathing when I can't sleep.
- I had trouble emptying the dishwasher because it was difficult to put the dishes on the shelf that was too high, so I changed the kitchen cabinets, and I bought some drawers so that I can put things away while sitting down. This allows me to save energy to do other things that I like. Despite the vertigo, I signed up for a group dance class.
- I discovered that it makes me feel good to take at least ten minutes in the evening to sit on the couch. You have to learn to stop and dedicate time to yourself. In the end, we have to be the most important people on earth for ourselves, so we have to love ourselves.
- Coming here helped me learn to ask for help and I saw that people are willing to help.
- Break down big goals into small goals, so they are more achievable and I have less anxiety.
- Being able to prioritize, there are obstacles and habits that prevent you from reaching your goal, you have to "take steps to clear the way": for example, I spend too much time dusting, so I decided to remove several objects that I don't actually need and so I spent much less time.
- When I feel like I can't do it, I sit down.
- I don't pick up the baby when I have to bathe her because she weighs twenty kilos. I ask my husband to do it. I don't go to the park with the girls today if I can't do it, but maybe I'll do it tomorrow.
- I plan activities, I optimize my energy, but now I have to balance the rest activities. Before I always denied myself this, now I need it and I stop for a moment to catch my breath. I experience this as a transitory situation and I would like to have a legal right to be able to take my recovery minutes, I need legitimacy. I have always asked a lot of myself, I have always had great expectations and I also have to be able to justify to myself this "slowing down". The fact of being here is something that shows that I put myself on the line and that I took a space just for myself. When I come to the meetings it is regenerating for me and gives me energy for the following weeks.
- I realized that in addition to physical fatigue, I need to manage mental fatigue, so it helps me a lot to write down some things on my phone and "download a lot of information from my memory". Using aids like crutches is certainly a difficult step to take, but you have to realize when they are necessary. They help you have a freedom that you otherwise wouldn't have. To make my mother understand this, the doctor told her: "Just as if someone can't see they wear glasses, if they have difficulty walking they use supports".
- I try to plan activities and improve the environment. I used to be very messy, now I'm trying to create more order, even mentally, by establishing priorities in the things I have to do. I also try to stop in time when I start to feel tired.

- I overdo it with rest. Sometimes I do less than I actually could do, I should be a little more active.
- Maybe there is work to be done with regards to priorities, because sometimes I give priority to the wrong things and then it is more difficult to recover. My priority now is well-being and trying to find a balance between work, family and home.
- I am the exact opposite of everything, I am almost ashamed. There is never balanced rest with activity: I only stop when I lie down, maybe that is also why I sleep badly. I should give myself different rhythms, it is as if I were pretending not to be sick.
- Doing relaxation exercises at home I realized that the most tense area of my body is the jaw, I had never noticed it before.
- I have set priorities. At work, I have forced myself to sit down every now and then. At home, I have to give myself half an hour of rest otherwise I won't make it to the end of the day. With regard to the environment, I have tried to improve it with things that help me relax (blue lights, music…) and with aids such as the dishwasher.

Fourth meeting – Emotions, sensations, thoughts

Comments on negative, illusory and positive thoughts

- I go through periods: with multiple sclerosis I had an initial negative approach, then an illusory one, in which I deluded myself into thinking I had accepted it, and then a positive one, even though I haven't gotten there completely yet. It's useless to delude myself into thinking you've accepted the disease, if that were the case I wouldn't be here. I feel like I'm not going back, but that I am moving forward toward the positive, even though it's difficult to always have these thoughts.
- When I have to have an MRI I'm anxious until I get in, then I close my eyes and imagine singing little songs with my girls. I did the same during the lumbar puncture and it worked, it calmed me down.
- Sometimes when I drop something I immediately think of multiple sclerosis: in the immediate I feel bad and react, but then I justify myself by falling slightly into an illusory thought, as I can't find concrete elements of the manifestation of the disease.
- It is an objective problem to break a plate, but I identify with the "If I organize myself I can do it": I believe that if you look at life smiling, life smiles at you, you don't have to focus on the negative aspects but accept the change and adapt.
- I tend to be negative, this is due to many combined factors. I don't understand what I can do to get out of this vicious circle. With work, I've always been someone who, when faced with unfair criticism, said "Who cares": I have difficulty agreeing with my boss on the timing of doing the work, when I do things I want to do them well and if I have too little time I can't. I try not to care but in the end I do. I'm always angry and now I'm fed up. I'm a person who has always let arguments go, but inside I'm churning out anger.
- At the time of diagnosis and when I wasn't well, I saw myself thinking negatively. But since I've started therapy, I oscillate between positive and illusory thinking.
- For me, positive thinking should generate positive feelings, but thinking that I can still do certain things doesn't generate any of this, because before it was obvious that I could do them.
- Working at a bar, I often break plates or glasses and at first I think it's because of the illness, but then I see the other bartender who breaks even more than me and he's not ill. I'm aware of the fact that I broke some because I couldn't hold them in my hand but oh well, never mind.

Rules for managing negative emotions

- I use breathing a lot even if now I "practice" especially when I'm not very anxious because I'm not very good at it yet. In the evening, I almost always take ten to fifteen minutes to do a bit of yoga and relax; lately I've accompanied these moments with classical music by Einaudi and… it works!

- I'd like to let go of control a little: I always want to be in control of everything! This obsession with control also leads me to constantly search for a cause and it happened that I found myself asking myself, if this illness came to me because I did something wrong, because I didn't "let go" of many things… then rationality returns and the thought goes back in.
- Sometimes I found myself wondering if it was my character's fault, the fact that I'm an anxious person, the fact that I didn't let many things slide off of me… and often the people around me provoke these thoughts.
- What I realized is that it is necessary to "re-calibrate" oneself with respect to one's limits of the new condition: you have to observe yourself and understand how far you can go. It is clear that something has changed, that some things tire us more but perhaps we just need to reduce a little and not cancel everything or exclude everything a priori.
- I focused on the breathing that I practice before sleeping. I continue to be an insomniac, but if despite everything I continue to do it is because it gives me something positive.
- Negative thinking kills you; illusory thinking eludes reality, eludes the problem; therefore, it can be dangerous because it leads you to act inconsiderately. And if one does not act consciously you can fail and therefore fall into the negative.
- I try to relax with my breathing in moments when I am not particularly agitated about learning; I look for situations that are positive and fun for me and I listen to music that calms me down.
- I pay attention to my body to understand how to manage my energies, but I practically don't talk about it with anyone because those close to me will never be able to fully understand… in fact… when I hear advice (which often seems like reprimands) from those close to me (friends, mother…) I perceive them negatively and therefore I withdraw and avoid discussion again.
- After all, they will never be able to truly understand what my emotions are and what I feel; but if I talk to others who have multiple sclerosis or to you who are professionals, I am willing to listen, and I also take the "reprimands" more positively… healthy people cannot understand what I really feel!
- I recognize myself quite a bit in positive thinking, but when I am quite sad I tend to use illusory thinking, to avoid negative thinking. However, when it comes to doing things I find myself more in illusory thinking, because thinking "The important thing is that I did it, I do it as best I can" is depressing, it seems to me like saying that I will never be able to do that thing in a normal way. I see it as a defeat. I think I can do everything as well as before, maybe in a different amount of time but equally well.
- Before coming to these meetings, I characterized myself by illusory thinking and I never talked about the disease. Coming here and being "forced" to talk about it, I thought about it a lot more and I am slowly moving toward positive thinking. With respect to the last point, however, I find myself more in negative

thinking. It bothers me when the people I have told about the disease look at me, because it seems like they do it with pity or curiosity. In respect of not being able to do certain things, I cannot understand how much is due to the disease and how much to my will. However, the type of thinking also changes depending on the scope. With respect to university, I have seen an evolution from negative to positive thinking, with respect to physical activity I have not yet managed to make the transition to positive thinking. I am very uncompromising in the expectations, I have toward others and I am really angry with all those who do not have the disease. This thing is degenerating, because I extend this anger and intransigence to situations that have nothing to do with the illness.

- I asked myself why this happened to me, but I am trying to appreciate many more things than before.
- With respect to the illusory thought, it came to mind when in the first meeting I said that "thanks" to the disease I have the possibility of recreating myself. Instead, I find myself in the negative thought "I can no longer do this activity as well as before". I still try to commit myself, but I don't have the expectation of being able to do things as before.
- These meetings have helped me relax with my breathing and this helps me sleep and prepare for situations that I know could cause me anxiety.
- I have started listening to music again. Since I received the diagnosis I have stopped thinking about the past, while before I was a bit obsessed with it, I was attached to memories and gave them too much weight. This is a positive aspect.

Fifth meeting – communication

Comments on the topics of the fifth meeting

- Relationships with others are stressful, I hate it when they pity me, as if they had to take this moral weight off my shoulders; everyone advises me on what to do about my illness, and then, they feel sad, thus making me feel pitied.
- I am still me, beyond my difficulties, I have no serious physical problems, but every day is not the same; it is difficult to convince my husband that I am not already in a wheelchair. He is pessimistic, when usually I am. I wish everyone would stop pitying me for something that I don't even know what it is, if not a very heavy burden.
- It all seems like an exaggeration to me: everyone asking me how I'm doing when before they didn't care.
- I feel like I have to be well for others. I feel "guilty" because I "ignore" the symptoms and the disease itself that I don't know; my husband, on the other hand, worries too much, searches on the Internet, gets information. The disease has not only affected me, but my whole family.
- I am intolerant of my mother who seems more worried than me, she makes me feel "sick".
- I haven't told everyone that I have multiple sclerosis, because I don't want to see compassion in other people's eyes.
- I feel annoyed because friends who know I have multiple sclerosis, when they ask me how is it going, without calling my illness by name, but say "That something over there".
- I feel intolerant toward colleagues who have an attitude of flattery ("How you did that job, no one is capable").
- Colleagues ask how it is, without ignoring that I have multiple sclerosis but without making me feel "sick".
- I am able to self-determine, others (parents, but also friends) tend to make a sick person look infantile, others cannot know what we need, perhaps we have to educate them; I have to understand the sense of limit; sometimes there is also conflict with others.
- My partner has been very close to me, he has suffered with me. My parents always want to accompany me to visits, help me, but I don't always accept their help because I need to prove to myself that I can do everything on my own like before. My dad, even though he is present and available, I don't think he has yet fully understood what this disease entails, he is experiencing it like the flu, he thinks I will get better. He has always been like this, pretending not to see things and that problems don't exist, in general. My partner's parents treat me differently than before and it's something I can't stand. Those around me are having different reactions and I'm trying to orient myself.
- I don't like asking for help either, I prefer to be the one to help others. To be able to accept this situation I put myself in their shoes, if someone wants to help me it is right that I let them do it, for example I see that my sister cares about doing something for me and so I decided to get help with simple things, I do it both for her, so she feels useful, but also for me.

Follow-up meeting – 6 months after the course

Examples of what was useful and utilized in the group journey

- Breathing exercises were used to help me fall asleep. I thought a lot about using aids and I started delegating a lot, especially at work: I lost in salary but gained a lot in health. And I prefer it that way.
- I found the WhatsApp group very useful: we exchanged messages a few times to ask each other for advice.
- I tried to follow the rules for managing symptoms and to do more physical activity. I still feel the symptoms but I perceive them differently: I still struggle, but I feel better.
- Everything is fine, the illness was an excuse to do other activities that I didn't do before. For example, I just returned from a cruise with my parents, an experience I had never had.
- I focused on illusory, negative and realistic thoughts. I realized that I was only oscillating between negative and illusory. Life can go on. This was a small mental revolution.
- As I said before, the comparison in the group was particularly useful for me. Communicating with them was important.
- The fact of asking for help struck me. At first it weighed on me, I became grumpy when they offered me help. Then, I understood that it is important to communicate because sometimes what you think does not correspond to what the other person thinks or understands. I also talk to my son.
- I was afraid of going on vacation, but it went well and I learned to delegate more to my husband.
- I dwell on the here and now. I often wander with my mind, but it is important to stop because you miss things or worry about something that is not there yet.
- When I received the invitation I thought it was time to talk to someone about the disease. I know that the comparison is not always pleasant, but I wanted to try. So taking action is important, I have certainly strengthened my inner balance.
- The first meeting was a question mark, when I arrived here I thought: "but who made me do it" I was very skeptical, but now I have to say that I am satisfied.
- It helped me to put some fixed points in my life; I understood that I could still work and the group encouraged me to try and throw myself in. I re-evaluated my priorities and even at home I feel better. Now I am working, I take care of a baby of a few months and I also do another activity, I don't know where I find all this energy.
- As for relationships, I told my mother that I am sick, I didn't tell her that I have multiple sclerosis, I tried to let her know in a nice way and I simply said that it is a chronic disease. At work when I am sick I stop for a moment, I take my space and my time. In my free time I have dedicated myself to two physical activities.
- The best thing was meeting people like you. At first I was hesitant, I thought "I already have my sadness and do I have to feel the depression of others too?" Actually, it wasn't like that I only have certain conversations with them. It would be nice if it didn't end because it's good. I imagine it could also be positive for someone who is lonely, very depressed, who maybe thinks about suicide. Every

now and then I engage in breathing exercises, especially when I can't sleep. I need breathing, I really get into it.

- At first, I was very skeptical, but then through the group experience I no longer felt alone.
- Before, I was very detached from my emotions, with this path I got closer to this aspect, even if it was very tiring for me, I always thought that emotions can be something that hurts, that you have to distance yourself from.
- It is very tiring to reflect on yourself, on your life, but it is really useful.
- Sharing, for sure, because at the beginning of the illness I didn't even want to talk about it. It is difficult for me to get my emotions out, and sharing them in a neutral environment was definitely useful. These meetings also helped me understand that you have to focus on the present, while before I was totally worried about the future. Now I am managing to make short-term plans and focus more on daily activities.
- Sharing the problem. Before, there was only you – without terms of comparison and a comparison with others. For example, seeing that someone experiences the moment of the injection less negatively than you can help you put it into perspective.
- For me, it was important to reflect on my old and new needs, and discover my resources. It also helped me a lot to address the issue of communication with healthcare professionals. It helped me understand that if the doctor tells me that a symptom is normal, it is not to belittle it.
- Learning to ask for help is something I had never considered before.
- Being with people your own age helps one to bring out some things, because you can talk about aspects we have in common and compare yourself on multiple perspectives.

Observation grid of group meetings

Group Identifier: _____ Date: _____

_____ Start Time: _____

Meeting N°: _____ Ending Time: _____

Total Participants: _____ Observer: _____

Presentation of participants

→ Group arrangement: Indicate the arrangement of participants by writing an acronym for each of them (e.g., name initials).

_____

→ Report in summary what each participant said:

Participant 1	
Participant 2	
Participant 3	
Participant 4	
Participant 5	
Participant 6	
Participant 7	
Participant 8	

Summary of the content emerged

→ A summary report of what each participant said:

_____
_____
_____

Non-verbal behavior

→ Indicate for each participant the tone of the interventions made:

_____

→ Indicate the prevalent posture of the participants and significant changes in posture:

_____

→ Indicate the prevalent direction of the participants' gaze (towards the facilitator, towards another, towards their own lap/on the ground, far away/outside/towards a horizon that isn't there):

_____

Concluding remarks

→ Describe the climate of the group (with particular attention to the predominant emotions that emerged):

_____

→ Indicate the three words perceived as most recurrent in the group discussion:

_____

Answer the following questions briefly.

✔ Does the meeting room have adequate characteristics of size, microclimate, ventilation, lighting and noise? Is the room aesthetically pleasing?

_____

✔ Does the group layout allow everyone to look at each other?

_____

✔ Does the group express energy? Who/how is able to stimulate the energy of the group?

_____

✔ Is the relational climate positive? Who/how is able to promote a positive atmosphere?

_____

✔ Is everyone adequately recognized in their needs/desires?

_____

✔ How are participants' proposals received?

_____

✔ Are the members available to declare their opinions/thoughts?

_____

✔ Are participants listening while everyone expresses their thoughts?

_____

Attitude of participants

→ Indicate the predominant attitude of participants during the meeting (collaborative, interested in the opinions of others, open to discussion, resistant, oppositional, polemical, etc.).

Participant 1	
Participant 2	
Participant 3	
Participant 4	
Participant 5	
Participant 6	
Participant 7	
Participant 8	

Participants' experiences of the group

→ Indicate for each participant to what extent the group is experienced as **an opportunity for growth** and **openness to change** based on the following indicators:

- *Not at all:* The participant does not intervene or intervenes in a polemical and oppositional way, little interest in others' opinions, posture is closed (e.g., arms folded).

- *A little:* Interventions are not numerous, mostly at the request of the facilitator (question/answer), fair attention to other participants, prevalent posture closed.

- *Quite a lot:* The participants intervene spontaneously, in a constructive way, good attention to other participants, prevalent posture open and relaxed.

- *A lot:* Numerous, coherent, constructive interventions, grasps and re-elaborates the discussion points of the facilitator, opens up to the group also with the narration of personal episodes and/or expresses having put into practice or having reflected on what was discussed in the group, good interaction with other participants, open and relaxed posture.

	Not at all	A little	Quite a lot	A lot
Participant 1	0	1	2	3
Participant 2	0	1	2	3
Participant 3	0	1	2	3
Participant 4	0	1	2	3
Participant 5	0	1	2	3
Participant 6	0	1	2	3
Participant 7	0	1	2	3
Participant 8	0	1	2	3

→ For each participant, indicate to what extent the group is experienced as a **threat** and activates **resistance** based on the following indicators:

- *Not at all:* No difficulty in intervening and talking about oneself, does not demonstrate distance towards the facilitator or towards the other participants, open posture.

- *A little:* The participant intervenes little, sometimes if urged by the facilitator, quite willing to grasp the points of discussion as well interacts with other participants, predominantly open posture.

- *Quite a lot:* Interventions are quite few, struggles to express personal opinion, not willing to grasp what is said by the facilitator or the other participants, predominantly closed posture.

- *A lot:* The participant remains silent for most of the time and/or intervenes in a polemical and oppositional way towards the facilitator and/or the other participants, not willing to engage with others, closed posture, lost and/or distant gaze.

	Not at all	A little	Quite a lot	A lot
Participant 1	0	1	2	3
Participant 2	0	1	2	3
Participant 3	0	1	2	3
Participant 4	0	1	2	3
Participant 5	0	1	2	3
Participant 6	0	1	2	3
Participant 7	0	1	2	3
Participant 8	0	1	2	3

Appendix 4

Me and my life

Questionnaire

This questionnaire aims to better understand the experience of people who live every day with multiple sclerosis. Only you can know it and that is why your cooperation and your answers are precious. This knowledge will be used to carry out actions to improve well-being and quality of life of people living with multiple sclerosis.

Therefore, we ask you to fill out the various parts of the questionnaire below, taking special care **not to leave out any questions**.

We remind you that the questionnaire is **anonymous** and under the current law the information you will provide us will be treated with the utmost confidentiality. This information will only be used for **research purposes** and processed in **aggregated form.**

We ask you to write a **secret code** following the given instructions; this will allow us to match this questionnaire to the next ones that we will ask you to fill out.

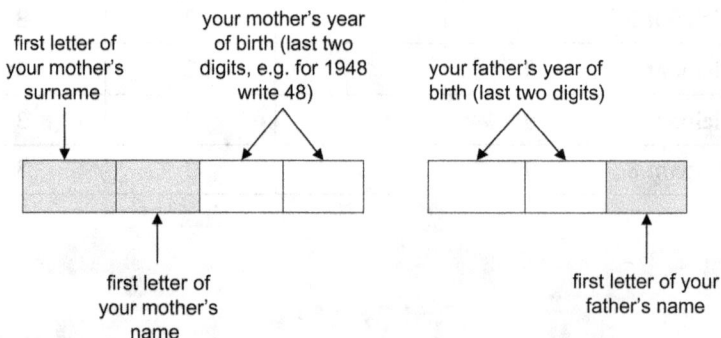

Your Secret Code

first letter of your mother's surname

your mother's year of birth (last two digits, e.g. for 1948 write 48)

your father's year of birth (last two digits)

first letter of your mother's name

first letter of your father's name

Date: ____/____/____

Let's start by asking you some personal data (put an **X** on the chosen square)

1 ☐ MALE   ☐ FEMALE

2 AGE _____

3 MARITAL STATUS:

   ☐ Unmarried   ☐ Married   ☐ Divorced/Separated

   ☐ Living with a partner   ☐ Widow

Have you got children?

☐ No   ☐ Yes   How many? _____   What's their age?_____

4 AT PRESENT, WHO ARE YOU LIVING WITH?

   ☐ alone   ☐ with children

   ☐ with husband/wife or partner   ☐ with parents

   ☐ with husband/wife or partner   ☐ other (please specify)_____
      and children

5 EDUCATION

   ☐ At least 8 years (middle school)

   ☐ At least 13 years (high school)

   ☐ More than 13 year (degree)

   ☐ other (please specify)_____

6 ARE YOU CURRENTLY DOING A PAID JOB?

   ☐ yes (please, go to question 9)   ☐ no (please, go to question 7)

7 HAVE YOU DONE A PAID JOB IN THE PAST?

   ☐ yes   ☐ no

8 HOW LONG HAVE YOU DONE A PAID JOB IN THE PAST?

   ☐ less than a year   ☐ for over 20 years

   ☐ for over a year   ☐ for over 30 years

   ☐ for over 10 years

9 When have you been diagnosed with multiple sclerosis? (year) _____

Please answer each of the questionnaire questions, as shown from time to time. If you don't feel certain about the answer, make the choice that seems better to you, without thinking about it too much. Remember that **there are no right or wrong answers**.

Let's start with some questions about your **health**.

10   In general, would you say your health is?

   ☐ Excellent   ☐ Very good   ☐ Good   ☐ Fair   ☐ Poor

11   The following items are about activities you might do during a typical day. Does your health now limit you in these activities? If so, how much?

		YES, limited a lot	YES, limited a little	NO, not limited at all
a.	**Moderate activities,** such as moving a table, pushing a vacuum cleaner, bowling or riding a bicycle	1	2	3
b.	Climbing **several** flights of stairs	1	2	3

12   During the **past 4 weeks**, have you had any of the following problems with your work or other regular daily activities as a result of your **physical health**?

		YES	NO
a.	Accomplished less than you would like	1	2
b.	Were limited in the kind of work or other activities	1	2

13   During the **past 4 weeks**, have you had any of the following problems with your work or other regular daily activities as a result of any **emotional problems** (such as feeling depressed or anxious)?

		YES	NO
a.	Accomplished less than you would like	1	2
b.	Didn't do work or other activities as carefully as usual	1	2

14 During the **past 4 weeks**, how much did **pain** interfere with your normal work (including both work outside the home and housework)?

☐ Not at all ☐ A little bit ☐ Moderately ☐ Quite a bit ☐ Extremely

15 These questions are about how have you felt during the **past 4 weeks**. For each question, please give the one answer that comes closest to the way you have been feeling. How much of the time during the **past 4 weeks**...

		All of the time	Most of the time	A good bit of the time	Some of the time	A little of the time	None of the time
a.	Have you felt calm and peaceful?	1	2	3	4	5	6
b.	Did you have a lot of energy?	1	2	3	4	5	6
c.	Have you felt downhearted and blue?	1	2	3	4	5	6
d.	Have you felt exhausted?	1	2	3	4	5	6

16 During the **past 4 weeks**, how much has your **physical health** interfered with your social activities (like visiting with friends, relatives, etc.)?

☐ Not at all ☐ A little bit ☐ Moderately ☐ Quite a bit ☐ Extremely

17 During the **past 4 weeks**, how much have your **emotional problems** interfered with your social activities (like visiting with friends, relatives, etc.)?

☐ Not at all ☐ A little bit ☐ Moderately ☐ Quite a bit ☐ Extremely

18 During the **past 4 weeks**, how much has your life been compromised by multiple sclerosis symptoms?

☐ Not at all ☐ A little bit ☐ Moderately ☐ Quite a bit ☐ Extremely

19 As a whole, how would you judge your quality of life? (put an **X** on the number that best represents your experience)

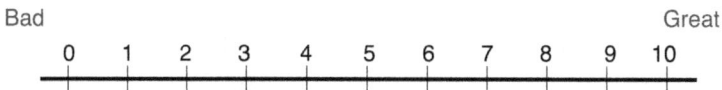

Bad   Great

0 1 2 3 4 5 6 7 8 9 10

20 Below is a list of the ways you might have felt or behaved. Mark how often you have felt this way during the past week.

1 = Rarely or none of the time	2 = Some or a little of the time (1-2 days)	3 = A moderate amount of the time (3-4 days)	4 = Most or all of the time (5-7 days)

a.	I was bothered by things that usually don't bother me	1	2	3	4
b.	I had trouble keeping my mind on what I was doing	1	2	3	4
c.	I felt depressed	1	2	3	4
d.	I felt that everything I did was an effort	1	2	3	4
e.	I felt hopeful about the future	1	2	3	4
f.	I felt fearful	1	2	3	4
g.	My sleep was restless	1	2	3	4
h.	I was happy	1	2	3	4
i.	I felt lonely	1	2	3	4
j.	I could not get "going"	1	2	3	4

21 Here is a series of questions relating to various aspects of your life. Each question has seven possible answers, with number 1 and 7 being the extreme answers. Please, circle the number which best expresses your feeling. Give only one answer to each question.

a. Do you have feeling that you don't really care about what goes on around you?

1	2	3	4	5	6	7
very seldom or never						very often

b. Until now your life has had:

1	2	3	4	5	6	7
no clear goals or purpose at all						very clear goals and purpose

c. Do you have the feeling that you're being treated unfairly?

1	2	3	4	5	6	7
very often						very seldom or never

d. Do you have the feeling that you are in an unfamiliar situation and don't know what to do?

1	2	3	4	5	6	7
very often						very seldom or never

e. Doing the thing you do every day is:

1	2	3	4	5	6	7
a source of deep pleasure and satisfaction						a source of pain and boredom

f. Do you have very mixed-up feelings and ideas?

1	2	3	4	5	6	7
very often						very seldom or never

g. Does it happen that you have feelings inside you would rather not feel?

1	2	3	4	5	6	7
very often						very seldom or never

h. Many people, even those with a strong character, sometimes feel like sad sacks (losers) in certain situations. How often have you felt this way in the past?

1	2	3	4	5	6	7
never						very often

i. When something happened, have you generally found that:

1	2	3	4	5	6	7
you overestimated or underestimated its importance						you saw things in the right proportion

j. How often do you have the feeling that there's little meaning in the things you do in your daily life?

1	2	3	4	5	6	7
very often						very seldom or never

k. How often do you have feelings that you're not sure you can keep under control?

1	2	3	4	5	6	7
very often						very seldom or never

We are interested in the expectations you have for the future: how do you see yourself at this stage of your life?

22 Here are some statements with which you may agree or disagree. Please indicate **how much you agree** with each statement, by putting an **X** on the number which best expresses your feeling.

1 = Absolutely disagree	2 = A little bit agree	3 = Quite agree	4 = Very agree	5 = Extremely agree

WHEN I THINK ABOUT MY FUTURE:

a.	I think I will feel useless and worthless	1	2	3	4	5
b.	I think I will feel unique	1	2	3	4	5
c.	I think I will feel unsure about who I am	1	2	3	4	5
d.	I think I will feel proud	1	2	3	4	5
e.	I think I will feel that my life is meaningful	1	2	3	4	5
f.	I think I will feel connected to my past	1	2	3	4	5
g.	I think I will feel isolated	1	2	3	4	5
h.	I think I will feel powerless	1	2	3	4	5
i.	I think I will feel capable and competent	1	2	3	4	5
j.	I think I will feel close to other people	1	2	3	4	5
k.	I think I won't be the same as before	1	2	3	4	5
l.	I think I will feel like any one	1	2	3	4	5

23   We now ask you to express your **satisfaction** with each of the areas listed below. Please, put an **X** on the number which best expresses your experience.

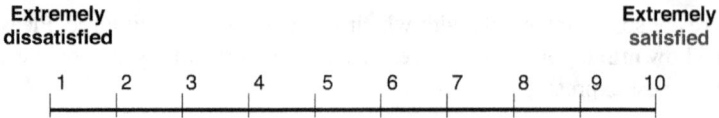

Extremely **dissatisfied**									**Extremely** **satisfied**
1	2	3	4	5	6	7	8	9	10

HOW SATISFIED ARE YOU...?:

a.	With your health	1	2	3	4	5	6	7	8	9	10
b.	With relationships with your friends	1	2	3	4	5	6	7	8	9	10
c.	With relationships with study or work colleagues	1	2	3	4	5	6	7	8	9	10
d.	With relationships with your family of origin	1	2	3	4	5	6	7	8	9	10
e.	With relationships with your current family (please, answer only if you no longer live with your family of origin)	1	2	3	4	5	6	7	8	9	10
f.	With relationships with your partner (please, answer only if you have a partner)	1	2	3	4	5	6	7	8	9	10
g.	With relationships with your children (please, answer only if you have children)	1	2	3	4	5	6	7	8	9	10
h.	With your study activities or job	1	2	3	4	5	6	7	8	9	10
i.	With your freetime activities	1	2	3	4	5	6	7	8	9	10

24   In general, how satisfied are you with your life? (please, put an **X** on the number which best expresses your experience)

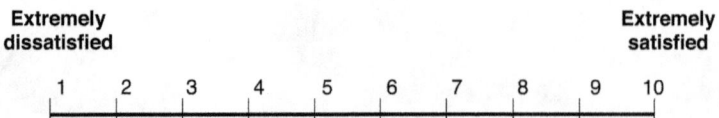

Extremely **dissatisfied**									**Extremely** **satisfied**
1	2	3	4	5	6	7	8	9	10

25   Here is a series of statements about situations that might be difficult to control. Please indicate **how much you feel confident** to deal with each situation, by putting an **X** on the number which best expresses your feeling.

1 = Not at all confident	2 = A little confident	3 = Quite confident	4 = Very confident	5 = Extremely confident

I AM CONFIDENT THAT I CAN:

a.	Take control over negative feelings (e.g., sadness, anger, anxiety)	1	2	3	4	5
b.	Organize the day and week time to reduce fatigue	1	2	3	4	5
c.	Find the way to do what it is important for me in the family	1	2	3	4	5
d.	Find the way to do what it is important for me in my job and social life	1	2	3	4	5
e.	Find the way to do what it is important for me with my friends	1	2	3	4	5
f.	Find the way to do what it is important for me during free time	1	2	3	4	5
g.	Setting new goals	1	2	3	4	5
h.	Find the way to reach goals	1	2	3	4	5
i.	Overcome the obstacles due to physical difficulties and disabilities	1	2	3	4	5
j.	Find the way to reduce the appearance and seriousness of physical disturbances	1	2	3	4	5
k.	Recognize what I can do in spite of physical limitations	1	2	3	4	5
l.	Not get discouraged because of unexpected events	1	2	3	4	5
m.	Search for support and help from others when I need it	1	2	3	4	5
n.	Voice my desires and preferences to family, friends, and colleagues	1	2	3	4	5
o.	Deal with day-to-day life in an autonomous way despite difficulties	1	2	3	4	5

26 Below you will find a list of adjectives that describe different **feelings and emotions**. Read each adjective carefully and see **how often** you experience each of them in **your daily experience**. Please, put an **X** on the number which best represents your experience.

1 = Never/almost never	2 = Few times	3 = Sometimes	4 = Many times	5 = Almost always/always

a.	Interested	1	2	3	4	5
b.	Distressed	1	2	3	4	5
c.	Excited	1	2	3	4	5
d.	Upset	1	2	3	4	5
e.	Strong	1	2	3	4	5
f.	Guilty	1	2	3	4	5
g.	Scared	1	2	3	4	5
h.	Hostile	1	2	3	4	5
i.	Enthusiastic	1	2	3	4	5
j.	Proud	1	2	3	4	5
k.	Irritable	1	2	3	4	5
l.	Concentrating	1	2	3	4	5
m.	Ashamed	1	2	3	4	5
n.	Inspired	1	2	3	4	5
o.	Nervous	1	2	3	4	5
p.	Determined	1	2	3	4	5
q.	Attentive	1	2	3	4	5
r.	Jittery	1	2	3	4	5
s.	Active	1	2	3	4	5
t.	Afraid	1	2	3	4	5

27 The following statements indicate possible ways to deal with **difficulties and problems** posed by multiple sclerosis. Please, tell us how many times **in the last month** you have happened to do or think about each of the things listed, by putting an **X** on the number which best describes your experience.

1 = Never	2 = Rarely	3 = Sometimes	4 = Often	5 = Very often

a.	I went on as if nothing happened	1	2	3	4	5
b.	I kept pushing myself to get things done	1	2	3	4	5
c.	I was able to express my emotions	1	2	3	4	5
d.	I concentrated my effort on things I can do	1	2	3	4	5
e.	I focused on the here and now	1	2	3	4	5
f.	I thought about how I might best solve the problem	1	2	3	4	5
g.	I talked to someone about how I felt	1	2	3	4	5
h.	I kept others from knowing my problems	1	2	3	4	5
i.	I couldn't express what I was feeling	1	2	3	4	5
j.	I tried to get something positive out of it	1	2	3	4	5
k.	I planned ahead what I needed to do	1	2	3	4	5
l.	I put it to the back of my mind	1	2	3	4	5

28 Finally, you will find some statements with which you may agree or disagree. Please indicate **how much you agree** with each statement, by putting an **X** on the number which best expresses your feeling.

1 = I strongly disagree	2 = I partially disagree	3 = I neither agree nor disagree	4 = I partially agree	5 = I strongly agree

		1	2	3	4	5
a.	In uncertain times, I usually expect the best	1	2	3	4	5
b.	It's easy for me to relax	1	2	3	4	5
c.	If something can go wrong for me, it will	1	2	3	4	5
d.	I'm always optimistic about my future	1	2	3	4	5
e.	I enjoy my friends a lot	1	2	3	4	5
f.	It's important for me to keep busy	1	2	3	4	5
g.	I hardly ever expect things to go my way	1	2	3	4	5
h.	I don't get upset too easily	1	2	3	4	5
i.	I rarely count on good things happening to me	1	2	3	4	5
j.	Overall, I expect more good things to happen to me than bad	1	2	3	4	5

29 Thinking about your current life, we now ask you to write what is the person or thing you rely most on.

_____

_____

_____

_____

_____

_____

Thank you for completing this questionnaire!

My point of view

Questionnaire

Please answer the questions below. They relate to the five group meetings that ended today. To answer please mark a cross (X) in the box that best expresses your opinion or use the lines to tell us your point of view. Please remember to fill in your secret code.

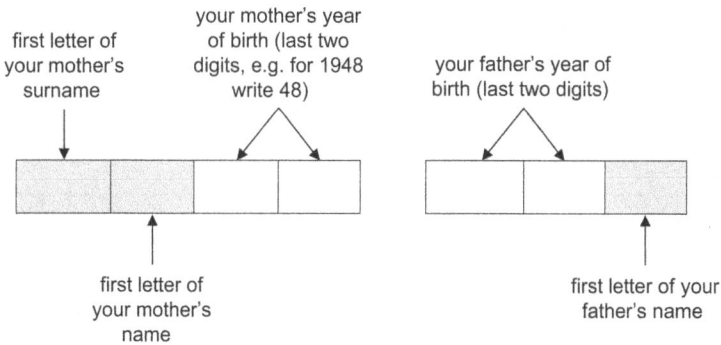

Your Secret Code

first letter of
your mother's
surname

your mother's year
of birth (last two
digits, e.g. for 1948
write 48)

your father's year of
birth (last two digits)

first letter of
your mother's
name

first letter of your
father's name

1 How do you rate the group experience you just completed?

☐ negative ☐ neither positive ☐ fairly ☐ positive ☐ very
   nor negative   positive   positive

2 Do you think this experience was useful for your life?

☐ not at all ☐ neither useful ☐ quite useful ☐ useful ☐ very useful
   useful   nor useless

3 Would you repeat this experience?

   ☐ yes   ☐ no   ☐ don't know

4 Would you recommend this experience to another person with MS?

   ☐ yes   ☐ no   ☐ don't know

5 Of this experience, what did you enjoy most?

   _____

   _____

   _____

   _____

   _____

6 Of the five meetings, which one did you enjoy the most?

   ☐ 1   ☐ 2   ☐ 3   ☐ 4   ☐ 5

7 Of this experience, what did you like least?

   _____

   _____

   _____

   _____

   _____

8 Of the five meetings, which one did you like the least?

   ☐ 1   ☐ 2   ☐ 3   ☐ 4   ☐ 5

9 Does it seem to you that something has changed in you since you started participating in the group?

   ☐ yes   ☐ no   ☐ don't know

10 If yes, did the change occur in a positive sense or in a negative sense?

   ☐ in a positive sense   ☐ in a negative sense

11   Was this experience tiring for you, mentally or physically?

☐ not at all   ☐ very little   ☐ somewhat   ☐ to a great extent

12   If you struggled, which encounter was most tiring for you?

☐ 1   ☐ 2   ☐ 3   ☐ 4   ☐ 5

13   Were you able to do the home exercises that were given to you from time to time?

☐ always   ☐ sometimes   ☐ occasionally   never

14   In conclusion, do you consider yourself satisfied with this experience?

☐ not at all   ☐ very little   ☐ somewhat   ☐ to a great extent

Thank you very much!
Your suggestions and evaluations will enable us to improve the program.

Appendix 6

Abstracts of published papers

For the reader's convenience, we provide below the abstracts of the scientific articles published by our working group. Readers interested in the full texts of the publications can find them through the bibliographic references provided.

Graziano, F., Calandri, E., Borghi, M., & Bonino, S. (2014). The effects of a group-based cognitive behavioral therapy on people with multiple sclerosis: A randomized controlled trial. *Clinical Rehabilitation, 28*, 264–274. https://doi.org/10.1177/0269215513501525

ABSTRACT

Objective. To evaluate the effectiveness of a cognitive behavioral group-based intervention aimed at reducing depression and fostering quality of life and psychological well-being of multiple sclerosis patients through the promotion of identity redefinition, sense of coherence, and self-efficacy.

Design. A randomized controlled trial.

Setting. Non-medical setting, external to the Multiple Sclerosis Clinic Centre.

Subjects. Eighty-two patients: 64% women; mean age 40.5, SD = 9.4; 95% with relapsing-remitting multiple sclerosis; Expanded Disability Status Scale (EDSS) between 1 and 5.5 were included in the study.

Interventions. Patients were randomly assigned to an intervention group (five cognitive behavioral group-based sessions, $n = 41$) or to a control group (three informative sessions, $n = 41$).

Main measures. Depression (CES-D), Quality of life (MSQOL revised), Psychological well-being (PANAS), Identity Motives Scale, Sense of Coherence (SOC), and Self Efficacy in Multiple Sclerosis.

Results. Quality of life increased in the intervention group compared with the control at 6-months follow-up (mean change 0.72 vs. −1.76, $p < 0.05$). Well-being in the intervention group increased for males and slightly decreased for females at 6-months follow-up (mean change 6.58 vs. −0.82, $p < 0.05$). Contrasts revealed an increase in self-efficacy in the intervention group at posttreatment compared with the control (mean change 2.95 vs. −0.11, $p < 0.05$). Depression tended to lower, while identity and coherence increased in the intervention group compared with the control, though the differences were not significant.

Conclusions. Preliminary evidence suggests that intervention promotes patients' quality of life and has an effect on psychological well-being and self-efficacy.

Calandri, E., Graziano, F., Borghi, M., & Bonino, S. (2017a). Improving the quality of life and psychological well-being of recently diagnosed multiple sclerosis patients: Preliminary evaluation of a group-based cognitive behavioral intervention. *Disability and Rehabilitation, 39*(15), 1474–1481. https://doi.org/10.1080/09638288.2016.1198430

ABSTRACT

Purpose. The study evaluated a group-based cognitive behavioral intervention aimed at promoting the quality of life and the psychological well-being of recently diagnosed multiple sclerosis (MS) patients (up to 3 years since the diagnosis).

Method. The study involved 85 patients [59% women; mean age 37, SD = 12.3; 94% with relapsing-remitting MS; Expanded Disability Status Scale (EDSS) between 1 and 4]. A quasi-experimental study design was applied; 54 patients (intervention group) participated in five group sessions, a 6-month post-intervention and a 1-year follow-up; 31 patients (comparison group) participated in activities routinely provided to recently diagnosed MS patients. Measures of Quality of Life (SF-12), Depression (CESD-10), Affective wellbeing (PANAS) and Optimism (LOT-R) were assessed.

Results. At the 6-month post-intervention, mental health increased in the intervention group and decreased in the comparison group, whereas negative affect decreased in the intervention group and increased in the comparison group. At the 1-year follow-up, mental health and optimism increased in the intervention group and decreased in the comparison group.

Conclusions. Preliminary evidence suggests that the proposed intervention fosters the quality of life and the psychological well-being of recently diagnosed MS patients by reducing negative affect and promoting mental health and optimism, particularly in the long term.

Calandri, E., Graziano, F., Borghi, M., & Bonino, S. (2017b). Coping strategies and adjustment to multiple sclerosis among recently diagnosed patients: The mediating role of sense of coherence. *Clinical Rehabilitation*, *31*(10), 1386–1395. https://doi.org/10.1177/0269215517695374

ABSTRACT

Objective. To examine the relationship between coping strategies (problem solving, emotional release and avoidance) and adjustment (health-related quality of life, depression and affective well-being) in a group of recently diagnosed multiple sclerosis patients (up to three years since diagnosis), and to explore the mediating role of sense of coherence between coping strategies and adjustment.

Design. Cross-sectional.

Setting. Multiple Sclerosis Clinic Centre.

Subjects. A total of 102 patients (61.8% women; age (years): M = 35.8, SD = 11.9; 95% with a relapsing–remitting form of multiple sclerosis; Expanded Disability Status Scale score, between 1 and 4).

Interventions. Not applicable.

Main measures. Coping with multiple sclerosis (problem solving, emotional release and avoidance), sense of coherence, health-related quality of life (SF-12), depression (CES-D) and affective well-being (PANAS).

Results. Problem solving was linked to higher mental health ($\beta = 0.28$) and higher affective well-being ($\beta = 0.36$), emotional release was related to lower depression ($\beta = -0.22$); avoidance was associated to higher mental health ($\beta = 0.25$), higher affective well-being ($\beta = 0.24$), and lower depression ($\beta = -0.29$) (all betas were significant at $p < 0.05$). Sense of coherence mediated the relationship between emotional release and depression (Sobel z-value = -2.00; $p < 0.05$) and the relationship between avoidance and all the indicators of adjustment (mental health: Sobel z-value = 1.97; depression: Sobel z-value = -2.02; affective well-being: Sobel z-value = 2.05; $p < 0.05$).

Conclusions. Emotional and avoidant coping strategies seem to be adaptive among recently diagnosed multiple sclerosis patients. A mediating role between coping strategies and adjustment is played by sense of coherence.

Borghi, M., Bonino, S., Graziano, F., & Calandri, E. (2018). Exploring change in a group-based psychological intervention for multiple sclerosis patients. *Disability and Rehabilitation*, *40*(14), 1671–1678. https://doi.org/10.1080/09638288.2017.1306588

ABSTRACT

Purpose. The study is focused on a group-based cognitive behavioral intervention aimed at promoting the quality of life and psychological well-being of multiple sclerosis patients. The study investigates how the group intervention promoted change among participants and fostered their adjustment to the illness.

Materials and methods. The intervention involved six groups of patients (a total of 41 patients) and included four consecutive sessions and a 6-month follow-up. To explore change, verbatim transcripts of the intervention sessions were analyzed using a mixed-methods content analysis with qualitative data combined with descriptive statistics. The categories of resistance and openness to change were used to describe the process of change.

Results. Resistance and openness to change coexisted during the intervention. Only in the first session did resistance prevail over openness to change; thereafter, openness to change gradually increased and stabilized over time, and openness to change was then always stronger than resistance.

Conclusions. The study builds on previous research on the effectiveness of group-based psychological interventions for multiple sclerosis patients and gives methodological and clinical suggestions to health care professionals working with multiple sclerosis patients.

Calandri, E., Graziano, F., Borghi, M., & Bonino, S. (2018). Depression, positive and negative affect, optimism and health-related quality of life in recently diagnosed multiple sclerosis patients: The role of identity, sense of coherence, and self-efficacy. *Journal of Happiness Studies*, *19*(1), 277–295. https://doi.org/10.1007/s10902-016-9818-x

ABSTRACT

The study aimed to describe the levels of depression, positive and negative affect, optimism and health-related quality of life (HRQOL) in a group of recently diagnosed multiple sclerosis (MS) patients (up to 3 years since the diagnosis), taking into account gender, age, and disease duration differences, and to investigate the possible role of identity, sense of coherence (SOC), and self-efficacy in MS (SEMS) on patients' depression, positive and negative affect, optimism, and HRQOL. The cross-sectional study involved 90 MS patients (61% women; age: M = 37, SD = 12) with an Expanded Disability Status Scale score between 1 and 4 (mild to moderate disability). Patients completed measures of depression (CESD-10), positive and negative affect (PANAS), optimism (LOT-R), HRQOL (SF-12), identity motives, SOC, and SEMS.

Depression scores were near the cut-off level for clinically significant depressive symptoms, and negative affect was higher and HRQOL was lower than those in the general population. Women and younger patients reported better adjustment as time passes since the diagnosis. Results of multiple regressions indicated that higher SOC was related to higher mental health, lower negative affect and lower depression. Higher SEMS was predictive of greater positive affect and lower negative affect, whereas higher identity satisfaction was predictive of higher positive affect and optimism and lower depression. The results suggest the usefulness of addressing identity redefinition, SOC and self-efficacy in psychological interventions aimed at promoting patients' adjustment to MS.

Bonino, S., Graziano, F., Borghi, M., Marengo, D., Molinengo, G., & Calandri, E. (2018). The self-efficacy in Multiple Sclerosis (SEMS) Scale: Development and validation with Rasch analysis. *European Journal of Psychological Assessment*, *34*(5), 352–360. https://doi.org/10.1027/1015-5759/a000350

ABSTRACT

This research developed a new scale to evaluate Self-Efficacy in Multiple Sclerosis (SEMS). The aim of this study was to investigate dimensionality, item functioning, measurement invariance and concurrent validity of the SEMS scale. Data were collected from 203 multiple sclerosis (MS) patients (mean age, 39.5 years; 66% women; 95% having a relapsing remitting form of MS). Fifteen items of the SEMS scale were submitted to patients along with measures of psychological well-being, sense of coherence, depression, and coping strategies. Data underwent Rasch analysis and correlation analysis.

Rasch analysis indicates the SEMS as a multidimensional construct characterized by two correlated dimensions: goal setting and symptom management, with satisfactory reliability coefficients. Overall, the 15 items reported acceptable fit statistics; the scale demonstrated measurement invariance (with respect to gender and disease duration) and good concurrent validity (positive correlations with psychological well-being, sense of coherence, and coping strategies and negative correlations with depression). Preliminary evidence suggests that SEMS is a psychometrically sound measure to evaluate perceived self-efficacy of MS patients with moderate disability, and it would be a valuable instrument for both research and clinical applications.

Calandri, E., Graziano, F., Borghi, M., & Bonino, S. (2019). Young adults' adjustment to a recent diagnosis of multiple sclerosis: The role of identity satisfaction and self-efficacy. *Disability and Health Journal*, *12*, 72–78. https://doi.org/10.1016/j. dhjo.2018.07.008

ABSTRACT

Background. Although multiple sclerosis (MS) is often diagnosed during young adulthood (18–30 years), there is a lack of knowledge on the psychological adjustment to the illness among recently diagnosed young adult patients.

Objective/hypothesis. The aims of the study were to describe the adjustment to MS (depression, positive and negative affect) in a group of young adult patients and to investigate the role of identity satisfaction and self-efficacy in MS on adjustment. We hypothesized that the relationship between identity satisfaction and adjustment was mediated by self-efficacy (goal setting and symptom management).

Methods. The cross-sectional study involved 66 patients (63.6% women) with a mean age of 25.2 years (SD = 3.4) who had been diagnosed for no more than three years. Patients completed measures of identity satisfaction (Identity Motives Scale), Self-efficacy in MS (SEMS), Depression (CESD-10), Positive and Negative Affect (PANAS). Data were analyzed through factorial ANOVAs and hierarchical regression analysis.

Results. Thirty-eight percent of patients reported depressive symptoms and negative affect mean score was higher than in the general population. Higher identity satisfaction was directly related to lower depression. Self-efficacy in goal setting partially mediated the relationship between identity satisfaction and positive affect, whereas self-efficacy in symptom management totally mediated the effect of identity satisfaction on negative affect. All results were significant at $p < 0.05$.

Conclusions. The results suggest the usefulness of addressing identity redefinition and self-efficacy in psychological interventions aimed at promoting young adults' adjustment to MS in an early phase of the illness.

Graziano, F., Calandri, E., Borghi, M., & Bonino, S. (2020). Adjustment to multiple sclerosis and identity satisfaction among newly diagnosed women: What role does motherhood play? *Women and Health*, *60*(3), 271–283. https://doi.org/10.1080/03630242.2019.1626789

ABSTRACT

The present study aimed to describe the levels of depressive symptoms, affective well-being and identity satisfaction in a group of women recently diagnosed with multiple sclerosis (MS), accounting for differences in age, motherhood, and disease duration. Moreover, the role of identity satisfaction in depressive symptoms and affective well-being was evaluated, examining the moderating effect of motherhood.

The study involved 74 women, aged between 19 and 57 years (Mean = 37.7 years, SD = 10.7 years). Thirty-two women (43.2%) had children, aged between 2 and 29 years. All women had relapsing-remitting multiple sclerosis (RRMS) and mild to moderate disability.

Mothers experienced greater depressive symptoms than childless women. Moreover, motherhood moderated the effect of disease duration on adjustment, with mothers reporting greater depressive symptoms, less affective well-being and less identity satisfaction than childless women as time passed since the diagnosis. Finally, greater identity satisfaction was related to less depressive symptoms and greater affective well-being, with a moderating effect of motherhood.

The results outline the relevance of the process of identity redefinition for women's adjustment to MS early in the illness. Moreover, the results underscore the need to take into account the additional burden of motherhood when promoting women's adjustment to MS.

Calandri, E., Graziano, F., Borghi, M., Bonino, S., & Cattelino, E. (2020). The role of identity motives on quality of life and depressive symptoms: A comparison between young adults with multiple sclerosis and healthy peers. *Frontiers in Psychology, Developmental Psychology Section*. https://doi.org/10.3389/fpsyg.2020.589815

ABSTRACT

The diagnosis of a chronic illness during young adulthood represents a non-normative life transition influencing the identity definition process, as well as the individual psychological adjustment. The study examined if relationships between identity motives (self-esteem, efficacy, continuity, distinctiveness, belonging, and meaning), health-related quality of life, and depressive symptoms differ between healthy young adults and young adults diagnosed with multiple sclerosis (MS). Two hundred one people (101 MS patients and 100 healthy controls), aged 18–35 years, completed a self-report questionnaire. Young adults with MS reported lower health-related quality of life and lower efficacy motive than their healthy peers. Among MS patients, high meaning was related to lower depressive symptoms, whereas high continuity and high belonging were related to higher health-related quality of life than in healthy controls. The study highlights the relevance of identity motives for the adjustment to MS and has implications for psychological interventions with young patients.

Calandri, E., Graziano, F., Borghi, M., & Bonino, S. (2021). The future between difficulties and resources. Exploring parents' perspective on young adults with multiple sclerosis. *Family Relations*, *71*(2), 686–706. https://doi.org/10.1111/fare.12630

ABSTRACT

Objective. To qualitatively explore parents' representations of the future of their young adult children diagnosed with multiple sclerosis (MS) and of their own future as parents.

Background. MS in young adulthood represents a nonnormative transition during the life cycle with a significant impact on the whole family. Previous research examined the perspective of parents having children and adolescents with MS, but there is a lack of knowledge about parenting young adults with MS.

Method. Thirteen semistructured interviews were conducted with parents of young adults (aged between 18 and 35 years) with MS, and an inductive content analysis was performed.

Results. The future of young people with MS in various domains (study, work and affective relationships) is deeply influenced by both illness and therapies. Parents' future is conditioned by the illness of their children. Family support and focusing on the present are recognized by parents as resources in coping with MS difficulties.

Conclusion. The uncertainty and unpredictability of MS influence parental representations of the future and represent an additional challenge in the difficult transition to adulthood.

Implications. The study gives indications for psychological interventions helping parents to cope with their children's illness and to stick to a personal future plan.

Graziano, F., Borghi, M., Bonino, S., & Calandri, E. (2024). Parenting emerging adults with multiple sclerosis: A qualitative analysis of the parents' perspective. *Journal of Child and Family Studies, 33,* 2367–2382. https://doi.org/10.1007/s10826-024-02845-8

ABSTRACT

Parents of emerging adults are requested to adjust their level of support and control according to their child's developmental age and to foster their autonomy. This developmental task may be more difficult when emerging adults are suffering from a chronic illness. Parenting emerging adults with a chronic illness is an under investigated topic, especially with reference to multiple sclerosis (MS), a chronic neurological disease usually diagnosed in emerging adulthood.

The study aims to qualitatively explore the characteristics of the relationship that parents report having with their emerging adult children (18–29 years) with MS. Specifically, we investigated how the dimensions of support and control emerge from the parents' perspective, whether overparenting (characterized by both oversupport and overcontrol) emerges, and its characteristics. Eleven semi structured interviews were conducted with parents of emerging adults with MS, and a qualitative content analysis was performed through Atlas.ti 6.0 software, combining a deductive and an inductive approach in relation to the study aims. A system of 13 codes was defined and a total of 141 quotations were codified.

Overparenting appears to be the most frequent relational mode among the parents interviewed. Most quotations referred to oversupport (in particular, parents report anticipatory anxiety about child's well-being and show excessive indulgence and permissiveness) and overcontrol (in particular, parents report a vicarious management of daily life and medical therapies). The study gives indications for psychological interventions helping parents to adequately support their children while encouraging their autonomous management of daily life and illness-related difficulties.

Graziano, F., Calandri, E., Borghi, M., Giacoppo, I., Verdiglione, J., Bonino, S (2025). Multiple sclerosis and identity: a mixed-methods systematic review. Disability and Rehabilitation, 47:9, 2199-2216. https://doi.org/10.1080/09638288.2024.2392039

ABSTRACT

Purpose. This systematic review addressed the following topics: (1) psychometric measures used to evaluate the identity/self in MS patients; (2) impact of MS on the identity/self of patients; (3) relationships between the identity/self and the adjustment to MS.

Method. Five electronic databases were searched for all peer-reviewed empirical studies published up to April 2024 (PROSPERO CRD42023485972). Studies were eligible if they included MS patients and examined identity/self through quantitative, qualitative or mixed-method study design. MMAT (Mixed Method Appraisal Tool) checklist was used to assess the quality of included studies. After conducting narrative synthesis (quantitative studies) and thematic synthesis (qualitative studies), an integration was undertaken following a convergent segregated approach.

Results. Forty-three studies were included (13 quantitative, 26 qualitative and four mixed methods). Studies used measures of "self" to refer to specific domains, and of "identity" to highlight the individual's uniqueness and continuity of experience over time. MS causes a loss of various aspects of self (physical, working, family and social self) and identity discontinuity. Maintaining a positive self-concept and integrating MS into one's identity are associated with better adjustment to MS.

Conclusion. Clinicians should consider the centrality of identity redefinition for the promotion of MS patients' adjustment to the illness.

Bonino, S., Calandri, E., Cattelino, E. (2025). Living with a chronic illness as a challenge to psychological development: The role of personal identity, sense of coherence and perceived self-efficacy, Social Sciences & Humanities Open, 11,101620 https://doi.org/10.1016/j.ssaho.2025.101620

ABSTRACT

The aim of this paper is to propose lifespan developmental psychology as a theoretical framework for analysing the psychological aspects of living with chronic illness. The basic assumption of lifespan developmental psychology is that development occurs throughout the entire human life-cycle. Furthermore, developmental psychology emphasizes the active role played by the individual in one's own development and pays particular attention to the adaptation processes involved. It underlines that development is prompted by challenging or crisis situations, provided that the person has the resources to deal with them. Based on these assumptions, chronic illness is considered not only as a constraint on development and a burden on existence, but also as a challenge that can promote psychological development: if illness undoubtedly entails considerable difficulties for personal development, it also has the potential to trigger transformation and positive adaptation processes. In this introductory theoretical article, we explain the model which we refer to and focus on three psychological variables, closely interrelated, that are crucial for adaptation to chronic illness: Personal identity, sense of coherence and self-efficacy. These aspects are particularly threatened by chronic illness, but also represent resources that can be strengthened and on which the person can count. We consider them key factors that can serve as resources in the process of personal development and adaptation to chronic illness throughout the lifespan. As examples, we report some of the results of our research on these aspects in people with multiple sclerosis. These findings confirm that it is useful to look at chronic illness from a developmental psychological perspective, not only for a deeper understanding of the processes involved, but also for the implementation of psychological support interventions.

Index

For Product Safety Concerns and Information please contact our EU
representative GPSR@taylorandfrancis.com
Taylor & Francis Verlag GmbH, Kaufingerstraße 24, 80331 München, Germany